# A Case-Based Approach
# to Public Psychiatry

CASE-BASED APPROACH SERIES

*A Case-Based Approach to Emergency Psychiatry*
Katherine Maloy

# A Case-Based Approach
# to Public Psychiatry

**EDITED BY**

**JEANIE TSE, MD**

CHIEF MEDICAL OFFICER, ICL, INC.

CLINICAL ASSISTANT PROFESSOR OF PSYCHIATRY

NEW YORK UNIVERSITY SCHOOL OF MEDICINE


**SERENA YUAN VOLPP, MD, MPH**

DIRECTOR, NYU PUBLIC PSYCHIATRY FELLOWSHIP

CLINICAL ASSOCIATE PROFESSOR OF PSYCHIATRY

NEW YORK UNIVERSITY SCHOOL OF MEDICINE

Oxford University Press is a department of the University of Oxford. It furthers
the University's objective of excellence in research, scholarship, and education
by publishing worldwide. Oxford is a registered trade mark of Oxford University
Press in the UK and certain other countries.

Published in the United States of America by Oxford University Press
198 Madison Avenue, New York, NY 10016, United States of America.

CIP data is on file at the Library of Congress
ISBN 978–0–19–061099–9

This material is not intended to be, and should not be considered, a substitute for medical or other
professional advice. Treatment for the conditions described in this material is highly dependent on
the individual circumstances. And, while this material is designed to offer accurate information
with respect to the subject matter covered and to be current as of the time it was written, research
and knowledge about medical and health issues is constantly evolving and dose schedules for
medications are being revised continually, with new side effects recognized and accounted for
regularly. Readers must therefore always check the product information and clinical procedures
with the most up-to-date published product information and data sheets provided by the
manufacturers and the most recent codes of conduct and safety regulation. The publisher and the
authors make no representations or warranties to readers, express or implied, as to the accuracy or
completeness of this material. Without limiting the foregoing, the publisher and the authors make
no representations or warranties as to the accuracy or efficacy of the drug dosages mentioned in the
material. The authors and the publisher do not accept, and expressly disclaim, any responsibility
for any liability, loss or risk that may be claimed or incurred as a consequence of the use and/ or
application of any of the contents of this material.

9 8 7 6 5 4 3 2 1

Printed by Webcom Inc., Canada

# CONTENTS

Public psychiatry encompasses the myriad behavioral health service delivery systems funded by government-sponsored health insurance and contracts—that is, the majority of psychiatric services provided internationally. As such, the vast majority of psychiatrists, whether or not they have received specialized public psychiatry training, are practicing public psychiatry. Included are psychiatrists working in city, state, and federal systems, nonprofit hospitals, community-based mental health or substance abuse agencies, and most academic centers. Only psychiatrists primarily working in private practices and, arguably, for-profit hospital systems are excepted.

In private practice, with patients who are financially secure, it is often possible to treat the person without much reference to the individual's environment. However, most people treated in public psychiatry settings need help to deal effectively with the systems that provide their primary and specialty health care, financial support, housing, education, employment, and social relationships.

The case studies that comprise this book exemplify how psychiatrists can help individuals navigate the systems with which they interact. Accordingly, these case studies are organized not as traditionally done by diagnosis but, rather, through a population health lens. These cases illustrate that public psychiatrists cannot operate in isolation. Rather, they need to be able to function flexibly in each of the four research-based roles identified by the Mental Health Services Committee of the Group for the Advancement of Psychiatry as defining systems-based practices: the roles of patient care advocate, team member, information integrator, and resource manager.

The health care system is in a rapid stage of transformation, accommodating emerging scientific findings, new clinical models, innovative technologies, and rising cost-control and quality requirements. Psychiatrists are increasingly expected to practice within a recovery model and to implement evidence-based interventions. Psychiatric education and mentoring at the residency, fellowship, and early career stages needs to equip psychiatrists with the concepts and skills to cope with this changing health care environment.

The research base necessary to guide trainees through the system's transformation is sparse. The existing literature is often written at a high level of abstraction that, although conceptually useful, provides little guidance to a recently graduated psychiatrist who gets a job at a community program embedded in a dense network of social service agencies. This book has been written with this clinician in mind, along with the many clinicians who provide public services in settings of unimaginable diversity. The psychiatric services of today have moved beyond the classic hospital-based community mental health center that dominated the last half of the 20th century. Today, there is astounding variation in governance, philosophy, and clinical approach.

The authors of this text, many veteran clinicians and/or founders of innovative public psychiatry programs, have wisely chosen a case-based approach. You can find here a powerful rendering of the many ways in which we fall ill in the 21st century; how culture, race, class, age, gender, and sexual orientation shape the clinical narrative; and how our social circumstances affect our health, access, and response to care.

It is a delight to immerse yourself, through this book, in the philosophical climate of public psychiatry. In some pages, you can feel the spirit of passionate advocacy that founded a program; in others, you hear the lyrics of community activism, the embrace of diversity, and the spirit of service. It is easy, through this book, to stand in awe and celebration of the commitment to heal people and communities that has animated contemporary psychiatry since the early days of the community mental health movement. This book may inspire you to serve, too.

Jules Ranz
Manuel Trujillo

The public perception of psychiatrists may still involve an image of a lone doctor in an office with a couch. However, today most psychiatrists have learned and practice psychiatry in environments that rely on public funding, working with some of the most socioeconomically disenfranchised people in our communities. This is not a job they do alone but, rather, in teams of behavioral health care workers and as part of larger health care and social systems.

During approximately the past 10 years, the number of public/community psychiatry fellowships has mushroomed from 2 programs to 17 today. This astonishing statistic reflects a growing recognition of the need for further training to provide principles and practices critical to the successful delivery of mental health care in an evolving health care environment. The editors and many of the chapter authors are faculty or alumni of these public psychiatry fellowships, and our aim with this book is to provide the next generation of public psychiatrists with a clinically oriented introduction to the skills and strategies we have found helpful.

The book first discusses seven principles with which every psychiatrist needs to be familiar—recovery, trauma-informed care, integrated care, cultural humility, harm reduction, systems of care, and financing care—using cases to bring these foundational concepts to life. Then, using a population health framework, cases are used to explore the typical needs of different groups and evidence-based/best practices to meet these needs. The second section sweeps "across the lifespan" from the needs of the very young to those of the very old. Some of the most compelling evidence supporting prevention work can be found in these chapters. We round out this section with a chapter on working with families, which is important with all age groups: Building an individual's natural support system is central to the recovery-oriented practice of psychiatry.

The third section shines a spotlight on specific populations that may have increased difficulty accessing care. Integrated, "one-stop-shop" care models figure prominently here as ways of overcoming access barriers. Cases illustrate the impact of the "deinstitutionalization" of mentally ill patients from state psychiatric hospitals in the 1960s and 1970s and the subsequent rise in the number of mentally ill individuals on the streets and in prisons; creative solutions to these issues are presented. Other vulnerable populations discussed include people with co-occurring substance use disorders, developmental disabilities or HIV, and people experiencing barriers to care due to migration, rural living, gender identity, or sexual orientation. Finally, programs for veterans are discussed, both because this population experiences unique challenges and because, as the only nationwide publicly funded health care system in the United States, the Veterans Administration presents a key case study in systems of care.

Some of the discussions regarding legal, financial, and structural aspects of care are skewed toward the current landscape in the United States because the "public" distinction is less significant in places with single-payer health care. However, we have kept the Canadian experience in mind, and we tried to make the discussion of treatment approaches universally relevant. We also acknowledge the varied use of "patient," "client," "consumer," "person served," and "individual" across behavioral health, and we have made no attempt to homogenize the use of these terms but instead have made a point of referring to our fictional characters by their names in the case histories.

Common to all the chapters is a focus on the potential of each person, regardless of illness, to achieve his or her personal goals, supported by a public psychiatrist armed with a knack for motivational interviewing and an advocacy bent. What will the next generation of public psychiatry innovations look like? We hope the readers of this book will be the architects of that future.

**Antonia Barba, LCSW**
Program Director
Bridging the Gap
Jewish Board of Family and Children's
Services
New York, NY

**Mary Barber, MD**
Clinical Director
Rockland Psychiatric Center
Associate Clinical Professor of
Psychiatry
Columbia University College of
Physicians and Surgeons
Orangeburg, NY

**Sonal Batra, MD**
Staff Psychiatrist
Princeton House Behavioral Health
Princeton, NJ

**Carissa Cabán-Alemán, MD**
Medical Director of Behavioral Health
Camillus Health Concern, Inc.
Assistant Professor
Department of Psychiatry and
Behavioral Health
Herbert Wertheim College of Medicine
Florida International University
Miami, FL

**Flavio Casoy, MD**
Chief Medical Officer
JSA Health California
New York, NY

**Jason Cheng, MD**
Associate Chief Medical Officer/Vice
President of Integrated Health
ICL, Inc.
Clinical Assistant Professor
New York University School of
Medicine
New York, NY

**Hilary S. Connery, MD, PhD**
Clinical Director
Alcohol and Drug Abuse
Treatment Program
McLean Hospital
Assistant Professor
Harvard Medical School
Boston, MA

**Jay Crosby, PhD**
Program Director
OnTrackNY@Bellevue
Bellevue Hospital Center
Clinical Assistant Professor
New York University School of Medicine
New York, NY

**Laura Erickson-Schroth, MD, MA**
Assistant Professor
Comprehensive Psychiatric Emergency
    Program
Mount Sinai Beth Israel
Psychiatrist
Hetrick–Martin Institute
Empowerment, Education & Advocacy
    for LGBTQ Youth
New York, NY

**Anita Everett, MD DFAPA**
President
American Psychiatric Association
    (2017–2018)
Arlington, VA
Associate Professor
Johns Hopkins Department of
    Psychiatry
Baltimore, MD

**Mia Everett, MD**
Director of Clinic Psychiatry
    Services
ICL, Inc.
New York, NY

**Elizabeth Ford, MD**
Chief of Psychiatry
Correctional Health Services
New York City Health + Hospitals
Clinical Associate Professor of
    Psychiatry
New York University School of
    Medicine
New York, NY

**Joanna Fried, MD**
Assistant Medical Director
Project for Psychiatric Outreach to the
    Homeless, Janian Medical Care
Medical Director
Manhattan Outreach Consortium
Clinical Instructor
New York University School of
    Medicine
New York, NY

**Ruth Gerson, MD**
Director
Child Comprehensive Psychiatric
    Emergency Program
Bellevue Hospital Center
Clinical Assistant Professor of
    Psychiatry
New York University School of
    Medicine
New York, NY

**Paulette Marie Gillig, MD, PhD**
Director and Professor
Division of Rural Psychiatry
Boonshoft School of Medicine
Wright State University
Dayton, OH

**Yu-Heng Guo, MD**
Psychiatrist
Corporal Michael J. Crescenz Veterans
    Affairs Medical Center
Clinical Assistant Professor of
    Psychiatry
University of Pennsylvania Perelman
    School of Medicine
Philadelphia, PA

**Alison M. Heru, MD**
Professor of Psychiatry
University of Colorado School of
    Medicine
Denver, CO

**Poh Choo How, MD PhD**
Assistant Clinical Professor
Department of Psychiatry and
    Behavioral Sciences
University of California, Davis School
    of Medicine
Sacramento, CA

**Larissa Lai, BA**
Evaluation Program Manager
Innovations Department
ICL, Inc.
New York, NY

**Stephanie Le Melle, MD MS**
Director of Public Psychiatry
    Education
Associate Professor of Clinical
    Psychiatry
Department of Psychiatry
Columbia University
New York, NY

**Pachida Lo, MD**
Staff Psychiatrist
Kaiser Permanente
Sacramento, CA

**Sheku Magona, MD**
Psychiatrist
Kirby Forensic Psychiatry
    Center
Assistant Professor
    of Psychiatry
New York University School of
    Medicine
New York, NY

**Rachel Mandel, MD**
Associate Director
Child Comprehensive Psychiatric
    Emergency Program
Bellevue Hospital Center
Clinical Assistant Professor of
    Psychiatry
New York University School of
    Medicine
New York, NY

**Marc W. Manseau, MD, MPH**
Associate Medical Director
Adult Services
New York State Office of
    Mental Health
Clinical Assistant Professor of
    Psychiatry
New York University School of
    Medicine
New York, NY

**Hunter L. McQuistion, MD**
Director
Department of Psychiatry & Behavioral
    Health
Gouverneur Healthcare, New York City
    Health+Hospitals
Clinical Professor of Psychiatry
New York University School of Medicine
New York, NY

**Leora Morinis, MA**
Medical Student
University of California, San Francisco
San Francisco, CA

**Paula Panzer, MD**
Chief Clinical and Medical Officer
The Jewish Board
New York, NY

**Ryan P. Peirson, MD**
Assistant Professor and Director
Division of Community Psychiatry
Chief of Forensic Psychiatry
Boonshoft School of Medicine
Wright State University
Dayton, OH

**Dennis Popeo, MD**
Unit Chief
Med/Geri Psychiatry Unit
Director of ECT Service
Bellevue Hospital Center
Director
Inter-clerkship Intensive
Associate Professor of Psychiatry
New York University School of Medicine
New York, NY

**Gertie Quitangon, MD, FAPA**
Director of Psychiatry
Community Healthcare Network
Clinical Assistant Professor of Psychiatry
New York University School of Medicine
New York, NY

**Jules Ranz, MD**
Director Emeritus
Public Psychiatry Fellowship
New York State Psychiatric Institute
Clinical Professor of Psychiatry
Columbia University College of
    Physicians and Surgeons
New York, NY

**Patrick Runnels, MD**
Director
Public and Community Psychiatry
    Fellowship
Director of Ambulatory Psychiatry
    University Hospitals
Medical Director,
The Center for Families and Children
Associate Professor
Department of Psychiatry
Case Western Reserve University
    School of Medicine
Cleveland, OH

**Anna Silberman, MS**
Masters in Neuroscience and Education
Columbia University Department of
    Psychiatry
Whitaker Developmental
    Neuropsychiatry Scholar
New York State Psychiatric Institute
New York, NY

**Stephanie Smit-Dillard, LCSW**
Clinical and Medical Services Division
The Jewish Board
New York, NY

**Sharon Sorrentino, PhD**
Vice President
Transitional Services
ICL, Inc.
New York, NY

**Michael Soule, MD**
Associate Director of Behavioral
    Health Integration
The Dimock Center
Roxbury, MA

**Shane S. Spicer, MD**
Assistant Professor of Clinical Psychiatry
Columbia University College of
    Physicians and Surgeons
Adjunct Professor,
New York University School of Medicine
Medical Director
The Lesbian, Gay, Bisexual and
Transgender Community Center
New York, NY

**Tara Straka, MD**
Psychiatrist
Kirby Forensic Psychiatric Center
Assistant Professor of Psychiatry
New York University School of
    Medicine
New York, NY

**Katharine Stratigos, MD**
Assistant Clinical Professor of Psychiatry
Columbia University Department of
    Psychiatry
Whitaker Developmental
    Neuropsychiatry Scholar
New York State Psychiatric Institute
New York, NY

**Nina Tioleco, MD**
Clinical Instructor in Psychiatry
Columbia University Department of
    Psychiatry
Whitaker Developmental
    Neuropsychiatry Scholar
New York State Psychiatric Institute
New York, NY

**Hendry Ton, MD, MS**
Interim Associate Vice Chancellor for
    Diversity and Inclusion, Associate
    Dean for Faculty Development and
    Diversity
Clinical Professor of Psychiatry and
    Behavioral Sciences
Director of Education
Center for Reducing Health Disparities
University of California, Davis School
    of Medicine
Sacramento, CA

**Manuel Trujillo, MD**
Director Emeritus
NYU Public Psychiatry
    Fellowship
Clinical Professor of Psychiatry
New York University School of
    Medicine
New York, NY

**Jeanie Tse, MD**
Chief Medical Officer
ICL, Inc.
Clinical Assistant Professor of
    Psychiatry
New York University School of
    Medicine
New York, NY

**Noah Villegas, MD**
Assistant Program Director
Rutgers New Jersey Medical
    School Residency Training
    Program
Clinical Instructor
Department of Psychiatry
Rutgers New Jersey Medical School
Newark, NJ

**Serena Yuan Volpp, MD, MPH**
Director
NYU Public Psychiatry Fellowship
Psychiatrist
NYC Department of Health and
    Mental Hygiene
Clinical Associate Professor of
    Psychiatry
New York University School of
    Medicine
New York, NY

**J. Rebecca Weis, MD**
Acting Medical Director and
    Consulting Psychiatrist
Early Childhood Mental Health
Mental Health Service Corps/ThriveNYC
Associate Director
NYU/Public Psychiatry Fellowship
Clinical Assistant Professor
New York University Department of
    Child and Adolescent Psychiatry
New York, NY

**Marjorie Westervelt, MPH**
Office of Medical Education
University of California, Davis School
    of Medicine
Sacramento, CA

**Agnes Whitaker, MD**
Clinical Professor of Psychiatry
Columbia University Department of
    Psychiatry
Research Psychiatrist
New York State Psychiatric Institute
New York, NY

**Erin Zerbo, MD**
Assistant Professor
Department of Psychiatry
Rutgers New Jersey Medical School
Newark, NJ

**Rachel Zinns, MD, EdM**
Chief of Outpatient Behavioral Health
Medical Director of Psychiatry
Westchester Medical Center
Assistant Professor
New York Medical College
Mount Pleasant, NY

# Foundational Principles

# Recovery Orientation as the Clinical Matrix

HUNTER L. MCQUISTION ■

## CASE HISTORY

Jay, 24 years old, unemployed since dropping out of high school, lives with his parents in a Midwestern town and is seen for an initial psychiatric evaluation. He presents as disheveled, saying he is "just about at the end of my rope," angry and depressed and constantly at odds with his parents. In a rambling way, he expresses suicidal thoughts, stating that for many weeks he has been ready to "snap at someone if they look at me the wrong way." Although never hospitalized, he vaguely speaks about past attempts at mental health care: "No one was interested in me." He smokes cannabis daily "to settle [his] nerves" and spends most of his time online browsing political websites and playing video games, unable to think about the future and goals, except for the desire to move out of his parents' house, with no clear idea of how to do so.

Jay feels alienated from people around him. He says that his parents and younger sister criticize and belittle him, and he believes that locals pick fights with him; he does all he can to avoid conflict. He complains of indistinct but disturbing hypnogogic visual and auditory hallucinations. Jay also has medical problems: chronic back and abdominal pains, epigastric distress, and, in passing, mentions that someone once said he might have liver disease, something called Wilson's.

### Clinical Pearl

### Recovery Orientation

Jay's problems are complex, and his sense of rage is concerning. But before discussing specifics, it is important to identify a powerful clinical approach that will assist him in overcoming his challenges and serve as an essential matrix in which clinical interventions are embedded—specifically, the paradigm of recovery orientation. During the past decade, the term *recovery orientation* has been increasingly conversant in behavioral health care and glimmering into the primary care mainstream. "Recovery" and "recovery orientation" have had an evolution of meaning and definitional variety (McQuistion & Sowers, 2014), but in order to best understand what follows, it is important to be clear:

> Recovery orientation embodies understanding how an array of practices can support people who are traveling through a uniquely personal and lifelong process that can be termed recovery, while also encouraging those who have not yet embarked on that journey and supporting them in the hope that they can do so. (p. 57)

Recovery is a journey. It can have endpoints, but it describes the narrative we build with our lives as we meet ongoing goals and challenges. It is a constantly unfolding process, yet nonlinear in nature. Recovery orientation in behavioral health focuses on assisting in that process, with clinical care as one of many tools a person employs in recovery. Although a psychiatrist may begin with a clinical approach, he or she will also purposefully assist a person to rely on and develop healing resources within occupational, recreational, kinship, friendship, spiritual, and other areas. This reaches beyond a more traditional biopsychosocial frame. For in-depth understanding, the reader may explore key foundational resources (Davidson, Rakfeldt, & Strauss, 2010; Ragins, 2002) and review the psychiatry Recovery to Practice curriculum, co-sponsored by the American Psychiatric Association and the American Association of Community Psychiatrists (American Psychiatric Association, 2015).

There are a number of crucial clinician attributes in recovery-oriented care, and they evolve as the relationship develops. They begin with fostering hope and consciously offering support of self-respect and self-determination, with an understanding that people must be in charge of their own wellness. Achieving this requires clinicians to focus on personal strengths, exercise empathic communication, be trauma-informed and culturally humble, proactively perform patient advocacy, and creatively use evidence-based practice. In addition, recovery orientation has important features of providing care that is comprehensive, coordinated, integrated, and, with rare exceptions, voluntary in nature.

In Jay's current situation, a conventional approach could be to take aggressive action with an impulsive, irritable, psychotic, and depressed person, who although in great pain—in fact, because of it—might need hospitalization to maintain safety and get a rapid start on accurate diagnosis and appropriate psychopharmacological treatment. However, you instead elected against hospitalization for the following reasons: You balanced a need for safety with the risk of a potentially traumatizing psychiatric hospitalization. Even in this first encounter, through connecting statements that focused less on symptomatology and instead on genuine interest in Jay's life, coupled with acknowledging courage in Jay's taking a risk to again seek help, Jay communicated desperate motivation to feel better. Over the course of 50 minutes, you recognized his sense of pain and frustration and explicitly stated that although professionals in the clinic are experts in mental health and its treatment, Jay is the expert on himself. You began to experience a sense of Jay's motivation to improve his situation even though he was somewhat disorganized in speech and behavior. At the end of the session, Jay agreed to return later the same week.

### Clinical Pearl

### Engagement Phase

The creation of a constructive relationship is time-honored in mental health care (Sullivan, 1954) but takes on new emphasis in recovery-oriented practice, with the patient recognized as being at the helm. This marks the initiation of a clinical stage that may be termed the *engagement phase* in the context of recovery orientation. *Motivational interviewing* (Miller & Rollnick, 2013) is a crucial tool to carry this forward. It honors a person's natural ambivalence about change, eliciting information with a preponderance of non-confrontational open-ended questions to identify ambivalence while supporting movement toward behavior change. It weaves in expressions of empathy and affirmation, and it focuses on what is important to the patient. These principles and techniques, as employed in recovery-oriented practice, are "person-centered" (Berwick, 2009), with historical antecedent in Carl Rogers' (1961) client-centered therapy.

Your engagement approach is to exhibit a serious attitude while communicating to Jay that the clinic will be equally serious in serving him. After identifying Jay's suffering with fear, anxiety, and frightening hallucinations, you offer to prescribe the antipsychotic aripiprazole. Jay is skeptical, saying "medication doesn't work." While bypassing debate on Jay's past medication adherence and balancing personal and community safety with treatment engagement, you specifically offer a low dosage and prompt follow-up. Responding to his skittishness about pharmacotherapy, you explain that it is important for both you and Jay to try a low dose to know if he tolerates the drug, leading to a discussion of side effects. This helps Jay's sense that his welfare and wishes are paramount.

Jay declines permitting you to contact his family, saying "they're not interested in therapy." You do not confront this at this time, even though engaging the patient's social network could be helpful. You then connect Jay with Sally, a psychotherapist on the clinic team who is adroit at case management. You emphasize to him that the team wants to offer as much support as needed.

### Clinical Pearl

### Collaboration

*Shared decision-making* (Center for Mental Health Services, 2010) is apropos of this interaction. This set of evidence-based techniques rests on having partnered conversations with a patient, arriving at person-centered goals that further an individualized treatment/recovery plan that the person owns. It assumes the presentation of a menu of intervention options—social, psychological, and pharmacological. For Jay, there was an agreement that his sense of irritability and impulsivity might improve with medication, which he was able to understand could be helpful. The next step is to begin to help him define some goals.

YOU: Where do you see yourself—what do you want to be doing—in, say, 2 years from now?

JAY: I want to move down to Colorado, where marijuana is legal.

A discussion about a means to support himself transpires, whether through work or disability benefits. The necessary step of financing any move is identified.

Clinical Pearl

Goal Setting

Breaking down larger goals to achievable objectives is a basic precept of psychi-atric rehabilitation (Liberman, 2008). But what happens when a patient wishes a clinician to do or not do something that may undermine his or her goals? One example is a person with a goal of sobriety who asks for indefinite treatment with benzodiazepines. In Jay's case, he declined to have the team reach out to family. While of course honored, the clinical team retained this as a possible future intervention. This highlights two important points. First, it underscores the need to fully clarify working goals in order to achieve progress, with the clinician supportively interpreting how granting some requests may be coun-terproductive. Second, a key principle of recovery orientation is that efforts to control are illusory and disempowering. Sometimes this effort derives from a sense of unrestrained responsibility for a patient's fate. Refraining from such behaviors liberates the clinician, enabling him or her to be the patient's trusted mental health expert. It is equally important to not translate this principle into a distortion of empowerment, with the clinician lapsing into doing what a patient wants at all times, thereby subverting true collaboration.

Over the course of several weeks, Jay discovers that "the pills help" and in fact self-titrates aripiprazole upward from 2 mg to 4 mg daily. You express appreciation about that information and acknowledge Jay's managing his own wellness. By now, Jay and the clinical team are seeking a better understanding of a now confirmed diagnosis of Wilson's disease, discussing the possibility that many of his psychiat-ric problems, including mood and psychotic experiences, are likely caused by that disease (Srinivas et al., 2008).

Subsequently, his meetings with the team are marked by periods of no-shows, coupled with exacerbations of irritability and the return of diffuse paranoid ide-ation. There is more than one episode of Jay raucously complaining about front desk staff—that they have "attitude" and do not meet his needs. His behavior evokes a sense of frustration—at times anger—on the part of his providers, especially when there is medication nonadherence and missed appointments with the hard-working team. Regarding missed appointments, it becomes clear that Jay has chal-lenges with memory and executive function, although a sense of pride restrained him from acknowledging it at first. Subsequent neuropsychological testing con-firms cognitive issues, now understood to be caused by Wilson's disease.

Clinical Pearl

Intensive Care Phase

The engagement phase segues into a phase termed *intensive care*, especially relevant in work with people with complex clinical presentations. This phase is marked by interdisciplinary interventions addressing sometimes rapidly evolving clinical issues that inform developing personal goals. Because of the potential for a multiplicity of issues, care must be taken to prioritize and clar-ify goals. There is ample opportunity to overwhelm the patient's resources, resulting in conflicts with staff, exaggerating transference and counter-transference phenomena. Jay's sensitivity to criticism by authority figures, combined with cognitive challenges, evokes rage against staff. Staff members' own anger could color their behavior—confrontation, coldness, or avoidance would be harmful.

Now approximately 9 months into their relationship, the team sets out with Jay to better understand his goals, meeting with him to prioritize how they could best be helpful.

Jay's stated goals are as follows:

1. Getting Social Security disability (SSD)
2. Scoring the right strain of weed ("*indica*—it's relaxing")
3. Avoiding conflict with parents
4. Moving to Colorado
5. Improving short-term memory

The following are the clinical team's concerns:

1. No income
2. Cannabis misuse
3. Inappropriate housing, with family conflict
4. Wilson's disease, with accompanying mental illness
5. Cognition: Difficulty managing a routine, short-term memory deficits

These lists are already fairly well aligned, and the following priorities arise (with an agreement to reassess in 3 months):

1. Work together on SSD. Although both Jay and his team believe it may not be needed permanently, this is vigorously pursued, with you and Sally both helping with appeals after initial rejection.
2. Take medication consistently. Psychoeducation is implemented to help Jay understand that his cognitive and mental health issues could be improved with appropriate chelation therapy for Wilson's disease, perhaps reducing the need for psychotropic medication. The team supports his efforts to keep track of medication.
3. Pursue cognitive rehabilitation, primarily to address Jay's embarrassing memory problems. He is introduced to Jim, a peer specialist at the clinic, who helps with appointment reminder calls and meets him for informal check-ins when Jay is at the clinic.

### Clinical Pearl

### Person-Centered Treatment Planning

A bulwark of recovery-oriented service is *person-centered treatment planning*. As opposed to traditional and mostly unilateral provider-driven treatment plans, this process requires active dialogue in planning, driven by the patient's goals. Adams and Grieder's (2013) work in this field describes a process of creating clinically useful treatment plans that articulate goals, barriers, strengths, realistically measurable objectives during a given time period, and interventions.

Therapy emphasizing cannabis misuse is not addressed at this phase of treatment planning. Jay's daily cannabis use likely hampers functioning, in a trade-off for his need to decrease anxiety, but the team elects to proceed only with educational forays, given his precontemplation stage of change within the transtheoretical model of substance misuse (Prochaska, DiClemente, & Norcross, 1992). It is also agreed that alternative housing be postponed until Jay has income.

### Clinical Pearl

#### Peer Supports

The meaningful integration of talents and skills of people who self-identify with lived experience with mental illnesses has gained important traction in service delivery (Repper & Carter, 2011). Peer workers act as liaisons to professionals, sometimes in an advocacy role. They are also uniquely qualified to interpret the meaning of treatment interventions to service users, especially when people are alienated from the service system. Integrating peer workers into the treatment team has several salutary purposes. First, in an in vivo manner, their presence educates professionals about patients' experiences, in fact helping service systems transform themselves—enabling systems to "recover" from archaic paternalistic models. Second, peer workers' transparency about having mental illnesses helps to destigmatize service users and increase self-confidence. Third, seeing a person with lived experience working and helping others inspires many patients to pursue their recovery.

About 2 months into Jay's intensive care, he phones you, saying "y'know, I think I should get a GED, can you help me with that?"

This was a watershed moment for Jay, heretofore living with a sense of desperate negative fatalism about his life. With Sally's help, he enrolls in a GED course and feels more in control of himself. He is coached in using a weekly medicine organizer, resulting in greater medication adherence. Also at approximately this time, he begins to consider how the clinical team could support him by meeting with his parents.

### Clinical Pearl

#### Ongoing Rehabilitation Phase

Although Jay is actively engaged in his recovery, he has yet to poise himself on a plane where mental health interventions become relatively de-emphasized and in which natural supports in work, housing, and love are predominant. This open-ended clinical phase is termed *ongoing rehabilitation*. In this phase, psychiatric care requires less activity due to a patient's greater ability for wellness self-management.

## DISCUSSION

The structural phases of clinical intervention and support noted in this chapter are engagement, intensive care, and ongoing rehabilitation (Figure 1.1). Although originally proposed for work with mentally ill homeless populations (McQuistion, 2012), they may be applied to others, especially when contextualized with the stages

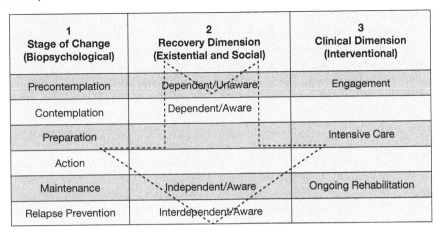

| 1<br>Stage of Change<br>(Biopsychological) | 2<br>Recovery Dimension<br>(Existential and Social) | 3<br>Clinical Dimension<br>(Interventional) |
|---|---|---|
| Precontemplation | Dependent/Unaware | Engagement |
| Contemplation | Dependent/Aware | |
| Preparation | | Intensive Care |
| Action | | |
| Maintenance | Independent/Aware | Ongoing Rehabilitation |
| Relapse Prevention | Interdependent/Aware | |

**Figure 1.1** Structural phases of clinical intervention and support.
SOURCE: From McQuistion (2012). Reprinted by permission.

of change (transtheoretical) model and with the dimensions of recovery (Townsend, Boyd, & Griffin, 2000). In the latter, a person moves from stark dependence on a system of care, "dependent but unaware" in the recovery journey, to become "interdependent and aware," understanding that people depend on each other to have optimal fulfillment and functioning. These three models align, as graphically described in Figure 1.1, with clinicians thinking interdimensionally and coordinating clinical interventions.

Importantly, recovery-oriented behavioral health interventions are consistent with evidence-based practice (Center for Medicare and Medicaid Services, 2015), such as peer support and motivational interviewing.

In fact, any credible clinical practice is recovery-oriented when it clearly serves a person's recovery goals. Although controversial, this may even include involuntary interventions that pursue personal and community safety. Behavioral health professionals, especially psychiatrists, have roles as agents of social control, complicating the person-centered precepts of recovery orientation. When thoughtfully considered, on a case-by-case basis, as ultimately serving a person's goals, inpatient and outpatient involuntary commitment honors recovery orientation. The key remains *always* keeping that human being who is—or you are striving to have as—your patient involved at the very center of any intervention.

## REFERENCES

Adams, N., & Grieder, D. M. (2013). *Treatment planning for person-centered care* (2nd ed.). Amsterdam, the Netherlands: Academic Press.

American Psychiatric Association. (2015). *Recovery to practice.* Retrieved from http://www.psychiatry.org/psychiatrists/practice/professional-interests/recovery-oriented-care/recovery-oriented-care-in-psychiatry-curriculum. Accessed November 27, 2015.

Berwick, D. M. (2009). What "patient-centered" should mean: Confessions of an extremist. *Health Affairs, 28*(4), w555–w565.

Center for Mental Health Services, Substance Abuse and Mental Health Services Administration. (2010). *Shared decision-making in mental health care: Practice, research, and future directions*. Rockville, MD: Author.

Center for Mental Health Services, Substance Abuse and Mental Health Services Administration. Practicing recovery: expanding person-centered care. Recovery to Practice Newsletter, Issue 2, April 2015. Available at http://ahpnet.com/Files/RTP-April-Newsletter-2015.aspx. Accessed November 28, 2015.

Davidson, L., Rakfeldt, J., & Srauss, J. (2010). *The roots of the recovery movement in psychiatry: Lessons learned*. Hoboken, NJ: Wiley-Blackwell.

Liberman, R. P. (2008). *Recovery from disability: Manual of psychiatric rehabilitation*. Washington, DC: American Psychiatric Press.

McQuistion, H. L. (2012). Homelessness and behavioral health in the new century. In H. L. McQuistion, W. E. Sowers, J. Ranz, & J. M. Feldman (Eds.), *Handbook of community psychiatry* (pp. 407–422). New York, NY: Springer.

McQuistion, H. L., & Sowers, W. E. (2014). Meetings minds on recovery: Why the time is now. *Journal of Psychiatric Administration and Management, 3*, 57–60.

Miller, W. R., & Rollnick, S. (2013). *Motivational interviewing: Helping people change* (3rd ed.). New York: Guilford.

Prochaska, J., DiClemente, C., & Norcross, J. (1992). In search of how people change: Applications to addictive behaviors. *American Psychologist, 47*, 1102–1114.

Ragins, M. (2002). *Road to recovery*. Los Angeles, CA: Village Integrated Service Agency. Retrieved from http://static1.1.sqspcdn.com/static/f/1084149/15460035/1323119957763/08ARoadtoRecovery.pdf?token=l3tKlYvFcSI%2BtqTdNcDtQZuqnZU%3D. Accessed November 27, 2015.

Repper, J., & Carter, T. (2011). A review of the literature on peer support in mental health services. *Journal of Mental Health, 20*(4), 392–411.

Rogers, C. R. (1961). *On becoming a person: A therapist's view of psychotherapy*. New York, NY: Houghton Mifflin.

Srinivas, K., Sinha, S., Taly, A. B., Prashanth, L. K., Arunodaya, G. R., Janardhana Reddy, Y. C., & Khanna, S. (2008). Dominant psychiatric manifestations in Wilson's disease: A diagnostic and therapeutic challenge. *Journal of the Neurological Sciences, 266*(1–2), 104–108.

Sullivan, H. S. (1954). *The psychiatric interview*. New York, NY: Norton.

Townsend, W., Boyd, S., & Griffin, G. (2000). *Emerging best practices in mental health recovery*. Columbus, OH: Ohio Department of Mental Health, Office of Consumer Services.

# Trauma-Informed Care

PAULA PANZER AND STEPHANIE SMIT-DILLARD ■

## CASE HISTORY

When we first meet Elle in the medical emergency room, she is an unemployed, 22-year-old, biracial mother of a 19-month-old boy. She resides with her boyfriend, the father of her son. She presents with abdominal pain and emesis. A psychiatric consultation is requested after Elle is told that her symptoms are due to pregnancy (estimated at 8 weeks), at which point she begins to cry in an uncontrollable fashion. Noticing the partially healed bruises on Elle's face, the staff nurse suspects domestic violence, but the medical resident "just doesn't believe it." When asked by the nurse, Elle states that she is "just clumsy" and ran into something. Elle leaves the emergency room with referrals and resources for maintaining a healthy pregnancy.

### Clinical Pearl

*Trauma* is defined as an experience that overwhelms an individual's ability to cope and elicits feelings of terror, helplessness, and/or out-of-control physiological arousal. Many people seeking help from health services have experienced emotional, physical, or sexual trauma that has direct bearing on their presenting symptoms but that often is neglected at key points of entry into the health care system. Use of routine, standardized trauma screening and assessment is an important part of patient care, regardless of an individual's initial explanation for his or her symptoms. By recognizing that traumatic experiences and their sequelae are closely intertwined with health and behavioral health symptoms, front-line practitioners can begin to build a trauma-informed system of care that provides the right treatment for the right symptoms.

Although guidelines indicate higher rates of identification of trauma exposure and accurate post-traumatic stress disorder (PTSD) diagnosis when evidence-based trauma screening tools are used (Substance Abuse and Mental Health Services Administration, 2014), best practice standards currently suggest a balance of structured questions and staff competency in a trauma-informed system of care.

In Elle's case, use of a validated screening tool to assess for the presence of intimate partner violence at the time she presents to the emergency room is a trauma-informed approach. Use of tools such as the Hurt Insult Threaten and Scream (HITS) screening tool (Sherin, Sinacore, Li, Zitter, & Shakil, 1998) or the Women Abuse Screening Tool (WAST) (Brown, Lent, Brett, Sas, & Pederson, 1996) and the use of compassionate, direct, open-ended questions are appropriate ways to understand the role of trauma in her presenting concerns. This screening should occur in a setting that maintains Elle's privacy and safety and should be accompanied by collaborative safety planning, including information for crisis services and supports, in light of her strong risk for re-exposure to violence. As with all services, Elle and others living with forms of violence must be permitted the dignity of choice in deciding what level of risk to safety they are willing to tolerate in their lives. The choice to pursue additional services or to seek out alternative living situations remains entirely with the patient, although in instances of reported child exposure to violence, child protective services must be consulted.

Two years later, Elle presents to a domestic violence (DV) shelter. She is still unemployed and now has two children and is almost 9 months pregnant. She fled her abusive boyfriend 3 months ago, and then she was forced to flee a DV shelter (where she initially sought refuge) when her ex was able to identify her location. Elle is deeply concerned about the safety of her children, and she worries that she will be found again.

Elle reports a relationship marked by financial control, demeaning language, isolation from family and friends, and recurrent physical and sexual violence. Her third pregnancy was the result of being raped by her boyfriend's brother. Elle's boyfriend blamed her for the assault in a graphic and degrading manner, and his family worked to ensure that Elle did not terminate the pregnancy or "give away" the child by keeping her under constant surveillance. She was eventually able to escape with her children to a shelter, where she proceeded with the pregnancy, fully intending to place the unborn child for adoption. She made all the agency contacts needed for this plan.

She describes a chaotic childhood, with physical abuse and neglect by her professionally employed, drug-dependent mother and sexual abuse (ages 7–12 years) by her mother's boyfriend. She reports that she did well in school but spent a lot of time with boyfriends, including in physically abusive relationships. She had mild affective dysregulation and some sleep disturbance as an adolescent but no marked losses of time or memory, flashbacks, self-harming, or suicidal behavior, nor drug or alcohol abuse. Elle states that she maintains contact with her mother for the sake of her 13-year-old half-sister, for whom she has ongoing safety concerns.

At the shelter, Elle presents with intrusive thoughts, nightmares, and hypervigilance, without flashbacks, isolation, somatization, despair, or suicidal ideation. She reports that she experienced flashbacks when she left her home. During the course of her 3-month stay at the first shelter, Elle was able to identify triggers for intrusive memories, and she learned to use relaxation techniques to calm herself so that the flashbacks subsided. She presented no overt conflict with the pending adoption plans and minimized the impact of her early life experiences on her current life.

## Clinical Pearl

Once patients screen positive for trauma, further assessment for trauma-related symptoms is necessary. Practitioners should expect avoidance from trauma victims in discussing their trauma histories due to feelings of shame or fear or avoidance of trauma triggers. These symptoms should be normalized and validated, without encouraging an overly detailed "spilling" of too much information too soon. Practitioners may unwittingly cause harm by moving too deeply or quickly into traumatic material without ensuring that patients have adequate coping supports and resources to manage their reactions. In general, practitioners should seek the middle ground between avoidance and oversharing by regularly checking in with the patient throughout the trauma assessment.

In Elle's case, the following domains of information are important to understand further:

- The impact of trauma on her physical health, including injuries, medical problems, pregnancy complications, hospitalizations, and access to care
- The psychological impact of the trauma, assessing for trauma-related symptoms aligning with DSM-5 trauma and stressor-related disorders as well as for symptoms of depression, anxiety, or serious mental illness
- The impact of the trauma on Elle's behaviors, emotional states, relationships, and level of functioning across settings in her life
- The effectiveness and safety of any coping strategies she currently uses
- The presence of strengths, skills, supports, resources, and resilience
- The presence of high-risk behaviors, suicidal thoughts including plan and intent, or impairment of parental functioning
- Potential re-traumatization in a shelter

Trauma survivors can show wide variations in how they experience and express traumatic stress reactions. Impairment or distress following trauma is mediated by multiple factors, including the nature of the trauma, the amount and duration of trauma experienced, individual history and attributes, developmental factors, sociocultural considerations, and available resources. Initial reactions to trauma exposure can include exhaustion, confusion, sadness, anxiety, numbness, dissociation, physical arousal, and blunted affect. Many of these responses are common and are socially acceptable, psychologically adaptive, and self-limited. Individual risk factors for developing PTSD include preexisting traits, including lower cognitive ability, negative cognitive bias, avoidant personality, and behavior problems, an existing personal trauma history and the absence of adequate social support (DiGangi et al., 2013; Haglund et al., 2007; Schoedl, Costa, Fossaluza, Mari, & Mello, 2014; Yehuda & LeDoux, 2007).

In Elle's case, additional information is required prior to making a differential diagnosis. Elle is currently experiencing intrusive thoughts, nightmares, and hypervigilance. Examples of validated measures for use in making a trauma-informed diagnosis include the Clinician-Administered PTSD Scale (CAPS; Blake et al., 1995) and the UCLA PTSD Reaction Index (Steinberg, Brymer, Decker, & Pynoos, 2004).

Co-occurence of PTSD with other mental health disorders, most commonly depression, substance abuse, and anxiety disorders, is as high as 80% by some estimates (Foa, 2009; Bradley et al., 2005).

Elle delivers a full-term baby girl, whom she names Chance, before placing her with adoptive parents at 2 days of age. Five weeks after delivery, Elle presents in acute distress. She experiences recurrent flashbacks of the abuse by her boyfriend and her parents. She is afraid of losing touch with reality because the old triggers for flashbacks (smells and sights) no longer seemed predictable. She has disturbances in sleep and appetite. In addition, she is overwhelmed by the new temper tantrums and separation anxiety in her 3-year-old child. Elle's son begins to ask if his younger brother will stay or go away. Elle believes that she is doing all that she can to take care of herself and her children and rages at the thought that no one ever did the same for her.

**Clinical Pearl**

Once Elle's trauma symptoms are better understood, it will be useful to expand the understanding of her trauma response beyond a diagnostic label and to consider her present difficulties from a resiliency perspective. This perspective views her symptoms as having once been normal, adaptive reactions to an unsafe environment. A key task of any trauma intervention is to support individuals in recognizing that trauma symptoms are no longer serving an adaptive purpose in the absence of any ongoing threats to their or others' safety. To this end, it is always important to understand the current level of safety for the patient in his or her community and also the stressors and mediators, including the social determinants of mental health that may impede recovery post trauma exposure.

Elle's children need to be considered in service planning because trauma can have far-reaching effects even on very young children. Children who experience threats to their own or to their caregiver's safety can develop challenges with emotional and behavioral regulation and may become clingy, fearful, or distrustful in the face of new people or situations. They may regress developmentally and may have difficulty self-soothing. Several evidence-based practices target trauma symptoms in children and families and are delineated further below.

## DISCUSSION

### Epidemiology

More than 75% of persons in the United States are exposed to at least one traumatic event in their lifetime (Breslau & Kessler, 2001; Kessler, Chiu, Demler, & Walters, 2005), with studies finding that repeated exposure to trauma is correlated with the emergence of significant health and mental health disorders later in life. Initial results from the Adverse Childhood Experiences Study (1998), jointly conducted by the Centers for Disease Control and Prevention (CDC) and Kaiser Permanente, show a strong and exponential correlation between the number of traumatic events encountered during childhood and adolescence and the emergence of problems in adulthood, including alcoholism, chronic obstructive pulmonary disease, ischemic heart disease, liver disease, and sexually transmitted disease.

Studies have also shown that childhood sexual abuse victims are more vulnerable to developing later physical and mental health challenges as well as sexual re-victimization (Black et al., 2011; Desai, Arias, Thompson, & Basile, 2002; Lalor & Mcelvaney, 2010). The CDC's "National Intimate Partner and Sexual Violence Survey (NISVS): 2010 Summary Report" (Black et al., 2011) found that more than one-third (35.2%) of the women who reported a completed rape before the age of 18 years also experienced a completed rape as an adult, compared to 14.2% of the women who did not report being raped prior to age 18 years.

## Interventions

Not every individual who has experienced trauma and is engaged in health or behavioral health services sees the need for, or wants, trauma treatment. For some patients, simply the idea of acknowledging trauma-related experiences may be too overwhelming, whereas others may engage in repeated, uncontrolled disclosure of the trauma before establishing a safe environment for developing coping skills. Trauma survivors will present with different levels of trauma awareness, urgency in need for trauma services, and readiness to engage with services. A provider's role is to help trauma survivors feel equipped to safely address trauma by developing adaptive behavioral and cognitive coping skills.

Trauma interventions occur on service and system levels. At a service level, treatment of trauma symptoms is often conceptualized as occurring in three phases: stabilization, resolution of traumatic memory, and integration. Phase 1 maintains a focus on ensuring patient safety, normalizing and validating trauma symptoms, providing psychoeducation, and assisting the patient in building skills for managing symptoms of physiological arousal that can accompany trauma cues. Phase 2 consists of exposure to traumatic material through imaginal or in vivo exposure, often entailing the writing of a trauma narrative. This phase usually employs cognitive processing to restructure maladaptive thoughts and beliefs related to the trauma. Personality integration and rehabilitation are the focus of phase 3. The goal is to help the patient return to fully functional daily living and enhance future safety.

There exists a great deal of evidence suggesting that cognitive–behavioral therapy (CBT) approaches to trauma are effective across a variety of populations in reducing PTSD and depression. CBT encompasses a range of short-term treatments that include both cognitive techniques (e.g., learning to think about something differently) and behavioral components (e.g., education and skill-building to put new thoughts into practice). Cloitre, Koenen, Cohen, and Han (2002) designed a sequentially based treatment for PTSD in adults that is organized into two phases: Skills Training in Affect and Interpersonal Regulation (STAIR), followed by the emotional processing of the trauma using a modified version of prolonged exposure, called Narrative Story-Telling (NST) or STAIR-NST. Their 2002 study found that STAIR-NST demonstrated improvements in affect regulation, interpersonal skills deficits, and PTSD symptoms.

For young children (ages 0–6 years), child–parent psychotherapy is a dyadic, relationship-based treatment that focuses on the way the trauma has affected parenting practices; the parent–child relationship; the intergenerational transmission of trauma; and the trauma's influence on the family's cultural values, spirituality, and beliefs (Cicchetti, Rogosch, & Toth, 2000; Lieberman, Ippen, & Van Horn, 2015). A caregiver's possibly maladaptive beliefs about the parent–child relationship, many of which may stem from a history of trauma or parental maltreatment, are explored and addressed.

For older children, adolescents, and young adults (ages 3–21 years), trauma-focused CBT (TF-CBT) addresses multiple domains of trauma, including PTSD, through a supported, gradual exposure approach (Cohen & Mannarino, 1997). TF-CBT engages children and a supportive caregiver in promoting skills for regulating affect, behavior, thoughts, and relationships; processing trauma; and enhancing safety, trust, parenting skills, and family communication. TF-CBT is supported by multiple randomized controlled trials showing improvements in a range of trauma symptoms.

Most clinical guidelines do not recommend pharmacological interventions as a first-line treatment for PTSD. However, medications such as selective serotonin reuptake inhibitors may be indicated when patients present with a sleep disturbance, when moderate/severe depression or hyperarousal interferes with the patient's ability to engage with or make gains in treatment, or when therapy alone has been found to be ineffective in reducing symptoms (National Institute for Clinical Excellence, 2005).

Based on the limited available evidence, it is recommended that patients with PTSD plus comorbid conditions be treated using a trauma-informed approach integrating components targeting specific co-occurring diagnoses (Bradley et al., 2005; Foa, 2009). Practitioners should take care when the presence of co-morbid psychotic symptoms indicates the use of specific therapies and anti-psychotic medication.

Beyond psychotherapeutic approaches, trauma victims often require significant care coordination and support in dealing with a myriad of pressing concerns, which may include dealing with ongoing issues of safety for themselves and their children, stabilizing their finances, acquiring new housing, or obtaining food. Without addressing these important instrumental needs, it can be challenging for trauma survivors to participate fully in therapy.

On a systems level, trauma-informed services espouse the belief that trauma can pervasively affect an individual's well-being. Trauma-informed providers are aware that patients with trauma histories may be more likely to experience treatment procedures as negative, reminiscent of past traumas, or dangerous and re-traumatizing. Practitioners should be collaborative and transparent in treatment to redress trauma survivors' histories of powerlessness, manipulation, and lack of control in decision-making. A trauma-informed system of care promotes the provision of safe, compassionate, collaborative care that recognizes and addresses the impact of trauma on patients while also supporting the staff who care for them.

The Sanctuary® model (Bloom, 1994, 1997, 2008) (an example of trauma-informed care) is a system-wide approach for organizational change that recognizes the parallel traumatization that can occur for both staff and patients in behavioral health care settings characterized by high trauma caseloads, significant resource constraints, and constant crisis response. These environments create a perceived lack of safety for staff and patients, and they can lead to organization-wide patterns of rigidity, suspicion, defensiveness, and combativeness that are like those exhibited by the patients whom the staff are attempting to serve. The Sanctuary®

model guides organizations to develop the following characteristics, promoting of trauma resolution:

- Nonviolence: Promoting safety for all
- Emotional intelligence: Teaching affect management skills to staff and patients
- Inquiry and social learning: Building cognitive skills
- Shared governance: Developing shared responsibility and healthy authority
- Open communication: Overcoming barriers to healthy communication
- Social responsibility: Rebuilding relationships
- Growth and change: Restoring hope, meaning, and purpose in the workplace

Creating a trauma-informed culture can result in less victim blaming, less punitive and judgmental responses from staff, and a better understanding of patients' treatment resistance or symptomatic behaviors.

Providers working with trauma survivors must be mindful of their own responses to traumatic material and attend to any emerging trauma-related symptoms in themselves. Working with trauma survivors can be overwhelming and exhausting, requiring providers to act as containers for highly distressing emotions and experiences. Referred to as secondary or vicarious trauma, a provider's trauma-related symptoms may interfere with the ability to effectively intervene with patients. A provider with a history of unresolved trauma, with significant stressors, or without adequate supports is particularly vulnerable to secondary trauma. The risk for secondary trauma is reduced when providers can receive training, consultation, and supervision in a collegial work environment, when they have the autonomy to pace their work and to take breaks, and when they can rely on adaptive coping strategies for identifying and reducing stress (Osofsky, Putnam, & Lederman, 2008). Most important, practitioners with an awareness of the far-reaching effects of trauma are best equipped to provide thoughtful, appropriate assessment and interventions in the service of their patients. With the support of a trauma-informed system, working with trauma survivors can be a deeply rewarding experience. Becoming a master over the trauma, rather than a victim of it, can often help a person enjoy life and function again, which can be overwhelmingly satisfying for the clinician who witnesses this transformation.

## REFERENCES

Black, M. C., Basile, K. C., Breiding, M. J., Smith, S. G., Walters, M. L., Merrick, M. T., ... Stevens, M. R. (2011). *The National Intimate Partner and Sexual Violence Survey (NISVS): 2010 summary report*. Atlanta, GA: National Center for Injury Prevention and Control, Centers for Disease Control and Prevention.

Blake, D. D., Weathers, F. W., Nagy, L. M., Kaloupek, D. G., Gusman, F. D., Charney, D. S., & Keane, T. M. (1995). The development of a clinician-administered PTSD scale. *Journal of Traumatic Stress, 8*, 75–90.

Bloom, S. L. (1994). The sanctuary model: Developing generic inpatient programs for the treatment of psychological trauma. In M. B. Williams & J. F. Sommer, Jr. (Eds.),

*Handbook of post-traumatic therapy: A practical guide to intervention, treatment, and research* (pp. 474–491).Westport, CT: Greenwood.

Bloom, S. L. (1997). *Creating sanctuary: Toward the evolution of sane societies.* New York, NY: Routledge.

Bloom, S. L., & Sreedhar, S. Y. (2008). The Sanctuary Model of Trauma-Informed Organizational Change. *Reclaiming Children and Youth, 17*(3), 48–53.

Bradley, R., Greene, J., Russ, E., Dutra, L., & Westen, D. (2005). A multidimensional meta-analysis of psychotherapy for PTSD. *The American Journal of Psychiatry, 162*(2), 214–227.

Breslau, N., & Kessler, R. C. (2001). The stressor criterion in DSM-IV posttraumatic stress disorder: An empirical investigation. *Biological Psychiatry, 50,* 699–704.

Brown, J., Lent, B., Brett, P. J., Sas, G., & Pederson, L. (1996). Development of the Women Abuse Screening Tool for use in family practice. *Family Medicine, 28*(6), 422–428.

Chan, A. O., & Silove, D. (2000). Nosological implications of psychotic symptoms in patients with established posttraumatic stress disorder. *Aust N Z J Psychiatry, 34,* 522–525.

Cicchetti, D., Rogosch, F. A., & Toth, S. L. (2000). The efficacy of toddler–parent psychotherapy for fostering cognitive development in offspring. *Journal of Abnormal Child Psychology, 28,* 135–148.

Cloitre, M., Koenen, K., Cohen, L., & Han, H. (2002). Skills training in affective and interpersonal regulation followed by exposure: A phase-based treatment for PTSD related to childhood abuse. *Journal of Consulting and Clinical Psychology, 70*(5), 1067–1074. doi:10.1037//0022-006X.70.5.1067

Cohen, J. A., & Mannarino, A. P. (1997). A treatment study of sexually abused preschool children: Outcome during one year follow-up. *Journal of the American Academy of Child and Adolescent Psychiatry, 36,* 1228–1235.

Desai, S., Arias, I., Thompson, M., & Basile, K. (2002). Childhood victimization and subsequent adult revictimization assessed in a nationally representative sample of women and men. *Violence and Victims Violence, 17*(6), 639–653.

Digangi, J., Gomez, D., Mendoza, L., Jason, L., Keys, C., & Koenen, K. (2013). Pretrauma risk factors for posttraumatic stress disorder: A systematic review of the literature. *Clinical Psychology Review, 33,* 728–744.

Foa, E. (2009). *Effective treatments for PTSD* (2nd ed.) New York, NY: Guilford.

Haglund, M. E. M., Nestadt, P. S., Cooper, N. S., Southwick, S. M., & Charney, D. S. (2007). Psychobiological mechanisms of resilience: Relevance to prevention and treatment of stress-related psychopathology. *Development and Psychopathology, 19,* 889–920.

Freuch, B. C., Grubaugh, A. L., Cusack, K. J., & Elhai, J. D. (2009). Disseminating evidence-based practices for adults with PTSD and severe mental illness in public sector mental health agencies. *Behavior Modification, 33*(1), 66–81.

Kessler, R. C., Chiu, W. T., Demler, O., & Walters, E. E. (2005). Prevalence, severity, and comorbidity of twelve-month DSM-IV disorders in the National Comorbidity Survey Replication (NCS-R). *Archives of General Psychiatry, 62,* 617–627.

Lalor, K., & Mcelvaney, R. (2010). Child sexual abuse, links to later sexual exploitation/high-risk sexual behavior, and prevention/treatment programs. *Trauma, Violence, & Abuse, 11*(4), 159–177. doi:10.1177/1524838010378299

Lieberman, A. F., Ghosh Ippen, C., & Van Horn, P. (2015). Don't hit my mommy!: A manual for Child-Parent Psychotherapy with young children exposed to violence and other trauma. Washington, DC: ZERO TO THREE.

National Institute for Clinical Excellence. (2005). *Post-traumatic stress disorder (PTSD): The management of PTSD in adults and children in primary and secondary care* (Clinical Guideline 26). London, UK: Author.

Osofsky, J. D., Putnam, F. W., & Lederman, C. S. (2008). How to maintain emotional health when working with trauma. *Juvenile and Family Court Journal, 59*(4), 91–102.

Schoedl, A., Costa, M., Fossaluza, V., Mari, J., & Mello, M. (2014). Specific traumatic events during childhood as risk factors for posttraumatic stress disorder development in adults. *Journal of Health Psychology, 19*(7), 847–857. doi:10.1177/1359105313481074

Sherin, K. M., Sinacore, J. M., Li, X. Q., Zitter, R. E., & Shakil, A. (1998). HITS: A short domestic violence screening tool for use in a family practice setting. *Family Medicine, 30*(7), 508–512.

Steinberg, A. M., Brymer, M., Decker, K., & Pynoos, R. S. (2004). The UCLA PTSD Reaction Index. *Current Psychiatry Reports, 6,* 96–100. Retrieved from http://springer.com/medicine/psychiatry/journal/11920

Substance Abuse and Mental Health Services Administration. (2014). *Trauma-informed care in behavioral health services: Treatment improvement protocol (TIP) series 57* (HHS Publication No. (SMA) 13-4801). Rockville, MD: Author.

Yehuda, R., & LeDoux, J. (2007). Response variation following trauma: A translational neuroscience approach to understanding PTSD. *Neuron, 56,* 19–32.

# Integrated Health Care

JASON CHENG AND JEANIE TSE ■

## CASE HISTORY

Wilma is a 43-year-old woman with schizophrenia who recently moved into a shelter near your clinic. Her auditory hallucinations have been well controlled with quetiapine 800 mg at bedtime. However, she gained 60 pounds after starting the quetiapine and became fatigued to the point where she was unable to maintain her cleaning job and could not pay her rent.

### Clinical Pearl

Psychiatric medications are among the factors that increase cardiometabolic risk among people with serious mental illness. Many psychiatric medications, including second-generation or "atypical" antipsychotics such as quetiapine, have metabolic side effects, including increased weight, glucose intolerance, and dyslipidemia. Screening guidelines provide the following recommendations (Vanderlip, Chwastiak, & McCarron, 2014):

- Medical history and waist circumference at baseline and annually thereafter
- Weight at baseline, then every 4 weeks for the first 12 weeks, then every 3 months thereafter
- Blood pressure, diabetes screening, and lipid panel at baseline, 12 weeks, and annually thereafter

Initiating treatment with a medication that has lower metabolic risk is good practice. For people who develop metabolic side effects with a medication that has been effective for psychiatric symptoms, the risks of switching medications should be weighed against the metabolic risks of the original medication.

Other factors increase the cardiometabolic risk for people with serious mental illness. Symptoms of mental illness, such as avolition and low energy, lead to reduced physical activity. Tobacco or substance use can also affect health (e.g., alcohol causing weight gain) and worsen self-care.

Communication between psychiatrists and primary care providers (PCPs) about management of metabolic side effects is important, but it does not always happen. Organizational solutions to communication issues are discussed later in this chapter.

Wilma has an elevated body mass index (BMI) of 31 and a waist circumference of 50 inches. You discuss the metabolic side effects of quetiapine, and she elects to switch to ziprasidone to reduce her risk. You e-mail her therapist Jose, your colleague at the clinic, about developing a plan for monitoring her symptoms, including safety risks. Jose confides that he is not accustomed to helping people with weight loss; you offer your support and a healthy living workbook you recently found. Jose and Wilma look at the workbook together, and she chooses to work on reducing sweets first.

Wilma says she had blood work at a primary care clinic recently and does not want to "be poked again." She signs a release of information form, and you fax it to the clinic. You do not hear back, so at the next appointment you call the clinic and a sympathetic receptionist faxes the results to you. The lipid profile is normal. Glucose was elevated, but Wilma says she had forgotten to fast.

### Clinical Pearl

Some people have difficulty fasting for blood work, but metabolic screening can still be done. Hemoglobin A1c is not affected by fasting state, so it can be used to screen for diabetes. Non-high-density lipoprotein (HDL) cholesterol varies by no more than 2% between fasting and non-fasting states. It is calculated by subtracting HDL from total cholesterol, and a value of 220 mg/dL or greater suggests dyslipidemia (Vanderlip et al., 2014).

You try to call the PCP who last saw Wilma, leaving messages without a return call. Wilma complains that the primary care clinic is far away, and she sees different staff every time she is there. You suggest she could see Dr. Augustin, who spends 1 day per week at your clinic as part of a new initiative. You are not at the clinic on the day Dr. Augustin is there, so you ask Jose to introduce Wilma to her.

Dr. Augustin orders a hemoglobin A1c, which is elevated. She recommends metformin and reinforces your recommendations for lifestyle change. However, Wilma has trouble meeting her health goals. She has been stressed out, and you explore the possible reasons. She says she recently began dating again, which has been triggering memories of childhood sexual abuse. You learn that when she is stressed, she tends to eat junk food and smoke cigarettes. You work with her to help her understand the link between her past trauma, current stress, and unhealthy behaviors.

### Clinical Pearl

Post-traumatic stress disorder is underdiagnosed, and the link between trauma and poor mental and physical health is often underappreciated. Reasons for this include lack of provider training, as well as both staff and patient discomfort with discussing trauma.

Broadly defined, trauma includes abuse, neglect, and household dysfunction. It is more prevalent in people who are homeless or have mental illness. The more types of trauma a person encounters during childhood, the higher the risk of mental illness. What may be more surprising is the higher risk of physical health issues as well, including obesity, heart disease, and chronic obstructive pulmonary disease (Felitti et al., 1998). This correlation may be mediated by unhealthy behaviors used to cope with post-traumatic symptoms such as anxiety. Trauma can also lead to mistrust, making engagement in treatment more difficult. A trauma-informed approach, discussed in the previous chapter, may lead to improved health behaviors.

Jose is also aware of the history of sexual abuse. Working with trauma is more familiar territory for him, and he finds it useful to think of Wilma's smoking as a maladaptive coping strategy. He says he will check in with her weekly regarding her progress on improving diet and physical activity. He will also follow up on whether she is attending appointments with Dr. Augustin.

### Clinical Pearl

An important aspect of treating any chronic condition is self-management, which involves individuals learning about their health conditions and how to manage them. Motivational techniques encourage individuals to discuss their goals and values, as well as changes they would like to make to achieve those goals. Individuals are supported in weighing the advantages and disadvantages of change. Readiness for change is assessed, and if there is enough commitment, individuals can choose specific, concrete, and achievable steps for change. Successful small steps generate momentum toward lasting change.

Wilma drinks three cans of cola per day and sets an initial action step to substitute water for one of these daily cans of soda. Wilma uses a log from the healthy living workbook to log her daily soda intake. After 2 months, she is not drinking any soda. She sets a new action step to walk around the block each day when she gets her mail. When she has a difficult time meeting this goal, you and Jose help her modify it and review the advantages and disadvantages of walking.

One action step at a time, Wilma improves her diet and increases physical activity. There are relapses—she has twice gone back to drinking soda, but she currently counts 38 "soda-free" days. After 6 months, her BMI decreases from 31 to 29. More important for her goal of returning to work, she has more energy. Jose helps her access a vocational program, and she finds a clerical job with a community agency. You discuss ways of staying physically active at a desk job.

She has achieved her goals in therapy, and you discuss whether she can continue obtaining ziprasidone from Dr. Augustin at the primary care clinic where Dr. Augustin works for most of the week rather than from you. Dr. Augustin has reservations about this, but you tell her you will be available to discuss Wilma's treatment and see her again if needed, and Jose will support care coordination.

## DISCUSSION

### Background

People receiving public mental health services die approximately 25 years younger than people in the general population (Lutterman et al., 2003). For people with schizophrenia, approximately 60% of premature deaths are due to treatable and preventable physical health conditions such as heart disease, stroke, and diabetes (Lambert, Velakoulis, & Pantelis, 2003). However, people with mental illness have poor access to treatment and poor quality of preventive care (Druss et al., 2010). These poor outcomes are associated with significant financial cost. People with disabilities, representing 15% of Medicaid beneficiaries, are responsible for almost half of the costs, spending approximately seven times as much as non-disabled adults, much of it from hospitalizations (Birnbaum, 2011).

At the same time, psychological trauma and depression often go undetected in the general population, leading to poor health outcomes. As many as 70% of visits to primary care sites "stem from psychosocial issues," and although "patients typically present with a physical health complaint, data suggest that underlying mental health or substance abuse issues are often triggering these visits" (Collins, Hewson, Munger, & Wade, 2010, p. 1). Both human and financial costs of a fragmented system have caught the attention of providers, regulators, and payers, leading to widespread efforts to integrate primary and behavioral health services.

### Models of Integrated Care

How is integration achieved? The four quadrant clinical integration model (Mauer, 2009) makes service recommendations for clients divided into four groups based on a two-by-two matrix by high or low level of behavioral health complexity and high or low level of physical health complexity. It recommends psychiatric consultation for populations with low behavioral health needs, such as those served by certain primary care clinics. For populations with high behavioral health needs, such as those served by specialty mental health programs, it recommends co-location of a PCP, and when the physical health need is also high, an additional nurse care manager is also recommended.

Providing behavioral health care in primary care settings is sometimes called "forward co-location," and the best-known model is collaborative care. In this model, PCPs screen people for mental illness, most commonly depression or anxiety. Those who screen positive can choose psychotropic medication prescribed by the PCP and/or brief, evidence-based psychotherapeutic interventions provided by an on-site behavioral health clinician. Both types of staff are supported by a consultant psychiatrist who is available to answer questions and who may also occasionally meet with patients to help direct care. Mental health symptoms are tracked regularly, with timely treatment adjustment for those who are not responding. More than 80 randomized controlled trials have been conducted on collaborative care, demonstrating improved depression and anxiety outcomes (Archer et al., 2012), improved outcomes in ethnic minorities (Interian, Lewis-Fernández, & Dixon, 2013), and cost-effectiveness in late-life depression (Unutzer et al., 2008).

One study demonstrated decreased cardiovascular events in older people with depression (Stewart, Perkins, & Callahan, 2014).

"Reverse co-location" puts primary care in the behavioral health settings in which people with serious mental illness are already engaged in care. Behavioral health counselors can have very close relationships with individuals, often seeing them more frequently than any other provider. Although the literature on reverse co-location is currently at a younger stage than that on forward co-location, there are nevertheless some promising research findings. On-site physical health interventions have been demonstrated to improve primary care linkage, rates of diagnosis of physical health conditions, and quality of physical health treatment for people with mental illness (Druss & von Esenwein, 2006).

Wilma's case illustrates that co-location of providers is key to integrating services. Communication is much easier when providers are just down the hall from each other. A trusted provider can use a "warm handoff" to a new provider to facilitate engagement. Shared health records and team meetings can also support coordinated care.

Co-location of all services is not possible. As such, care managers, whose specific role is to engage people in care and coordinate care across systems, are essential to support people with high needs. Care managers may be professionals, paraprofessionals, or peers (people with lived experience of mental illness). Care managers who do not have medical training will need supervision, education, and triage support, a role often fulfilled by nurses. Nurse care management, one of the recommended interventions for people with high behavioral and physical health complexity, can improve the quality of preventive health services (Druss et al., 2010). Nurses with both behavioral and physical health experience are particularly valuable to integration.

The four quadrant clinical integration model suggests that a continuum of services is needed. Ideally, people can move seamlessly from one level of service to another depending on the changing level of their behavioral and physical health needs. Current regulations requiring that mental health clinics admit and discharge people from care may present a barrier to continuity, as illustrated by questions about Wilma's disposition once her need for psychiatric services at the clinic ended.

## Psychiatry's Role in Management of Physical Health Conditions

Psychiatrists are experts in behavior change, which is fundamental to achieving better health outcomes; healthy eating, exercise, smoking cessation, and medication adherence are all behaviors. Using motivational enhancement techniques and trauma-informed approaches, psychiatrists can have a unique role in helping people manage cardiometabolic and other physical health conditions.

As described previously, metabolic side effects may warrant changes in psychiatric medications. In some situations, psychiatrists may also prescribe medications to address cardiometabolic risks, especially when clients are not engaged with primary care. For example, metformin, which is generally well tolerated and low risk, can be used to reduce weight in non-diabetic people with schizophrenia (Jarskog et al., 2013). Psychiatrists can also prescribe amlodipine for hypertension, statins for dyslipidemia, or aspirin to prevent heart attack if high risk, as the risk:benefit ratio for these medications is usually favorable and lab monitoring is simple.

There is a framework that can help evaluate when it is appropriate for psychiatrists to provide primary care interventions to people who have difficulty accessing adequate care (Vanderlip, Raney, & Druss, 2016). First, psychiatrists should consider urgency and complexity of the physical health problems. Routine, asymptomatic diabetes, hypercholesterolemia, and essential hypertension would be the most straightforward for psychiatrists to treat. Second, the poorer a client's access to primary care, the more appropriate it would be for a psychiatrist to treat routine physical health problems. Third, if a psychiatrist is knowledgeable and comfortable in treating certain physical health conditions, then doing so is within the psychiatrist's scope of practice. Availability of a PCP consultant is helpful although not required. Note that psychiatric nurse practitioners may not be able to treat physical health issues due to scope of practice limitations. Fourth, adequate systems should be in place for such tasks as collecting vital signs, tracking outcomes, and obtaining lab work. Finally, the client must of course agree to being treated by the psychiatrist. This framework is supported by and responds to the joint position statement of the American Psychiatric Association and the Association of Medicine and Psychiatry regarding the role of psychiatrists in addressing physical health disparities in patients with mental illness (Raney et al., 2016). To our knowledge, only one study (Golomb et al., 2000) has examined the expansion of a psychiatrist's role to include primary care interventions, and it found that a psychiatrist, supported by a primary care consultant, was an appropriate provider for most physical health conditions.

## Systems Challenges

Creating an integrated program involves hiring team members, designating and equipping spaces, designing workflows, and developing opportunities for communication and collaboration. The program's culture changes. If the licensing of a program changes, there may be a new set of regulatory requirements. Providers may not have the knowledge base for new tasks or may believe that new tasks are not their responsibility. It takes education and leadership to make integrated health a priority for an organization.

Financial sustainability may be another challenge. Depending on a program's regulations, integrated services may or may not be reimbursed. Generally, Federally Qualified Health Centers (FQHCs) are able to bill for primary care and behavioral health services in a more comprehensive way compared to community mental health centers. However, many FQHCs are not well equipped to care for people with serious mental illnesses, who may, for example, need psychosocial rehabilitation programs. Some behavioral health agencies have partnered with FQHCs to provide primary care services in a financially sustainable way. Integrated care has the potential to decrease utilization of expensive services such as emergency room visits and hospitalizations, so health care payers may be increasingly willing to pay for it.

Likewise, developers of electronic health records (EHRs) are addressing communication barriers between psychiatrists and PCPs, who have often used different

EHRs in the past. Ideally, all members of the integrated team will use the same record. At a minimum, providers must develop a system to exchange information, with a patient's consent. Health information exchanges and multiprovider treatment planning systems are becoming more common and can help providers integrate information about a person's care across programs.

Although integration poses a number of challenges, it has the potential to achieve the triple aim of improving the health care experience, improving population health, and reducing health care costs (Berwick, Nolan, & Whittington, 2008). Through both clinical and administrative roles, public psychiatrists can participate in this evolving integration.

## REFERENCES

Archer, J., Bower, P., Gilbody, S., Lovell, K., Richards, D., Gask, L., . . . Coventry P. (2012). Collaborative care for depression and anxiety problems. *Cochrane Database of Systematic Reviews, 10*, CD006525. doi:10.1002/14651858.CD006525.pub2

Berwick, D. M., Nolan, T. W., & Whittington, J. (2008). The triple aim: Care, health, and cost. *Health Affairs (Millwood), 27*(3), 759–769. doi:10.1377/hlthaff.27.3.759

Birnbaum, M. (2011). *Medicaid in New York: The road ahead.* New York, NY: Medicaid Institute at United Hospital Fund. Retrieved from http://www.medicaidinstitute. org/publications/880747. Accessed May 12, 2015.

Collins, C., Hewson, D. L., Munger, R., & Wade, T. (2010). *Evolving models of behavioral health integration in primary care.* New York, NY: Milbank Memorial Fund. Retrieved from http://www.milbank.org/uploads/documents/10430EvolvingCare/ EvolvingCare.pdf. Accessed May 7, 2015.

Druss, B. G., & von Esenwein, S. A. (2006). Improving general medical care for persons with mental and addictive disorders: Systematic review. *General Hospital Psychiatry, 28*(2), 145–153.

Druss, B. G., von Esenwein, S. A., Compton, M. T., Rask, K. J., Zhao, L., & Parker, R. M. (2010). A randomized trial of medical care management for community mental health settings: The Primary Care Access, Referral, and Evaluation (PCARE) study. *American Journal of Psychiatry, 167*(2), 151–159. doi:10.1176/appi.ajp.2009.09050691

Felitti, V. J., Anda, R. F., Nordenberg, D., Williamson, D. F., Spitz, A. M., Edwards, V., . . . Marks JS. (1998). Relationship of childhood abuse and household dysfunction to many of the leading causes of death in adults: The Adverse Childhood Experiences (ACE) Study. *American Journal of Preventive Medicine, 14*(4), 245–258.

Golomb, B. A., Pyne, J. M., Wright, B., Jaworski, B., Lohr, J. B., & Bozzette, S. A. (2000). The role of psychiatrists in primary care of patients with severe mental illness. *Psychiatric Services, 51*(6), 766–773.

Interian, A., Lewis-Fernández, R., & Dixon, L. B. (2013). Improving treatment engagement of underserved U.S. racial–ethnic groups: A review of recent interventions. *Psychiatric Services, 64*(3), 212–222. doi:10.1176/appi.ps.201100136

Jarskog, L. F., Hamer, R. M., Catellier, D. J., Stewart, D. D., Lavange, L., Ray, N., . . . Stroup, T. S.; METS Investigators. (2013). Metformin for weight loss and metabolic control in overweight outpatients with schizophrenia and schizoaffective disorder. *American Journal of Psychiatry, 170*(9), 1032–1040. doi:10.1176/appi. ajp.2013.12010127

Lambert, T. J., Velakoulis, D., & Pantelis, C. (2003). Medical comorbidity in schizophrenia. *Medical Journal of Australia, 178*(Suppl.), S67–S70.

Lutterman, T., Ganju, V., Schacht, L., Shaw, R., Monihan, K., Bottger, R., . . . Thomas, N. (2003). *Sixteen state study on mental health performance measures* (DHHS Publication No. (SMA) 03-3835). Rockville, MD: Center for Mental Health Services, Substance Abuse and Mental Health Services Administration.

Mauer, B. J. (2009). *Behavioral health/primary care integration and the person centered healthcare home.* Washington, DC: National Council for Behavioral Health. Retrieved from http://www.integration.samhsa.gov/Behavioral HealthandPrimaryCareIntegrationandthePCMH-2009.pdf. Accessed October 9, 2016.

Raney, L., Vanderlip, E., Rado, J., McCarron, R.; APA Workgroup on Integrated Care, APA Council on Healthcare Systems and Financing. (2016). *Joint APA/AMP position statement on the role of psychiatrists in reducing physical health disparities in patients with mental illness.* Arlington, VA: Fresno, CA: American Psychiatric Association/Association of Medicine and Psychiatry.

Stewart, J. C., Perkins, A. J., & Callahan, C. M. (2014). Effect of collaborative care for depression on risk of cardiovascular events: Data from the IMPACT randomized controlled trial. *Psychosomatic Medicine, 76*(1), 29–37. doi:10.1097/PSY.0000000000000022

Unutzer, J., Katon, W. J., Fan, M. Y., Schoenbaum, M. C., Lin, E. H., Della Penna, R. D., & Powers, D. (2008). Long-term cost effects of collaborative care for late-life depression. *American Journal of Managed Care, 14*(2), 95–100.

Vanderlip, E. R., Chwastiak, L. A., & McCarron, R. M. (2014). Integrated care: Nonfasting screening for cardiovascular risk among individuals taking second-generation antipsychotics. *Psychiatric Services, 65*(5), 573–576. doi:10.1176/appi.ps.201400015

Vanderlip, E. R., Raney, L. E., & Druss, B. G. (2016). A framework for extending psychiatrists' roles in treating general health conditions. *American Journal of Psychiatry, 173*(7):658–663. doi:10.1176/appi.ajp.2015.15070950

# 4

# Cultural Humility

CARISSA CABÁN-ALEMÁN ■

## CASE HISTORY

Imagine you are a consultation liaison psychiatrist, recently relocated from a rural clinic to a busy urban hospital. An obstetrician asks you to see Mrs. Santos, a 28-year-old Hispanic woman who just lost her newborn due to complications during delivery. She scored high on a standard postnatal depression scale.

Try to picture Mrs. Santos for a few seconds. What first came to your mind about her circumstances? Her appearance? What affect would you expect her to have? Do you expect her to be alone or accompanied?

### Clinical Pearl

In most instances, providers already have notions about a patient even before meeting him or her, just by knowing the patient's name, age, or address. Cultural humility begins when we recognize how our own cultures and assumptions influence the provider–patient relationship and, potentially, patient outcomes.

Before you go any further, briefly think about your own cultural background. Try to identify how it might be similar or different to Mrs. Santos' cultural values and how it might influence how you perceive her, as you read on.

You go to the nursing station to review Mrs. Santos' record, which only reveals that her postnatal depression score was 20. You cannot find the scale she completed. Her nurse, Ricky, approaches you and warns you that the patient is very angry. You ask him why she is upset, and he says he does not know—he is needed on another unit. What are your ideas about why she might be angry?

### Clinical Pearl

An initial interaction between a provider and a patient can be influenced not only by the provider's assumptions about the patient but also by the opinion of another professional and by dynamics between the patient and other team members. Being aware of this can reduce the risk of making biased or inaccurate conclusions when formulating an assessment and treatment plan.

You walk into Mrs. Santos' room, and she does in fact appear upset. You introduce yourself and state the reason why you are seeing her. She initially remains silent and does not respond to your questions, avoiding eye contact. You suspect she might not speak English and start thinking about calling an interpreter, but you ask her if she can understand English first. Suddenly, she yells, "Seriously? On top of the way that nurse treated us, now he sends me a shrink?!" Instead of proceeding to ask Mrs. Santos about the postnatal depression scale items or her recent loss, you say, "Tell me more about that." She reports that the nurse "had kicked out" her husband to take her vitals and give her the postnatal depression scale to complete. She states that she is angry because he did not let her husband return after visiting hours were over. Ricky also gave her a Spanish version of the postnatal depression scale. However, Mrs. Santos feels more comfortable reading English and is not fully fluent in Spanish. You apologize for what happened and tell her you wonder if the way she was feeling when completing the scale and the fact that she is not very comfortable with Spanish might have influenced the results. You ask Mrs. Santos if she could complete the scale again in English and she agrees. This time she scores a 12.

### Clinical Pearl

Patient-focused interviewing, as portrayed here, uses a less authoritative and controlling style that lets the patient know that the provider values the patient's perspective and is willing to focus on his or her agenda instead of the provider's priorities. This style creates an atmosphere in which the patient can give information about his or her beliefs to support the provider's assessment. This style also challenges power imbalances by empowering the patient to take on the expert role, as the provider becomes the student, learning about how the patient thinks and feels. Humility is necessary for the provider to be able to relinquish his or her usual role and offer a full partnership in the therapeutic alliance (Tervalon & Murray-García, 1998).

Language barriers can significantly impact the diagnostic assessment and treatment plan. With growing concerns about health disparities and the need for health care systems to accommodate increasingly diverse patient populations, language access services have become crucial for health care organizations. However, it is important to know when to use them—only if welcomed by, and not imposed upon, the patient.

Before discussing the situation with Mrs. Santos, you might have assumed that she was angry or lashing out, perhaps as a way of coping after her loss. Now that you have more information, you decide to discuss the issue with the nurse, attempting to avoid letting Mrs. Santos' negative opinion or physician–nurse power dynamics get in the way of understanding his perspective. Ricky tells you that he walked into Mrs. Santos' room yesterday to find a man dressed as a woman yelling "This is horrible!" in Spanish and crying. Concerned about the patient and her emotional state, Ricky asked him to wait outside while he took Mrs. Santos' vitals and asked her some questions. Mrs. Santos told him that her husband preferred to be called Sandy. Ricky shares with you that he felt extremely uncomfortable with the scenario and states, "I didn't know whether to call this man a he or she. I really did not expect that in a Hispanic family that just lost a baby." Ricky recently graduated from nursing school, and although he has lived in the city for years, he comes from a very conservative Latin family and has never met a transgender person before. Most of the normative cultural values he had learned to expect in Latinos did not match this scenario. He also took cultural competency training in which he was taught about what kind of cultural beliefs to expect from different ethnicities and how to use language services. He gave Mrs. Santos the Spanish version of the postnatal depression scale, hoping to be culturally competent, assuming that Spanish was her primary language because he heard her and Sandy speaking Spanish. However, he did not ask Mrs. Santos what language she preferred.

How would you have reacted if you were in Ricky's situation? Would you be comfortable with such a scenario? How would you have approached Mrs. Santos' husband?

### Clinical Pearl

Even when providers practice in a professional and humble manner, they might feel inadequate working with a patient who has cultural traditions or exhibits social constructs that they are not used to or might not agree with. Recognizing when this is the case is one of the first steps in cultural humility. The provider learns to avoid letting these feelings affect the development of rapport. Psychiatrists can avoid misdiagnosis and improve therapeutic effectiveness if they systematically assess how cultural factors influence diagnostic assessments (American Psychiatric Association, 2013).

You use some of the questions of the Cultural Formulation Interview from the DSM-5 to help you understand the context of Mrs. Santos' psychiatric symptoms and how she perceives them. You learn Mrs. Santos' mother is from Cuba. You might have assumed she is Latina from her last name. However, she is half Asian. She reports that she married Sandy very young. They started having issues last year when Sandy started to express her interest in becoming a woman. Soon after Sandy started the process of transitioning from male to female, Mrs. Santos became pregnant. Sandy feels guilty for the loss of the baby because of all the stress she put on Mrs. Santos, who had not been comfortable with Sandy's decision to transition, let alone with the financial cost. Sandy is also upset because she put hormone therapy on hold due to the pregnancy.

After Ricky reflects on the case, he decides to apologize to Mrs. Santos and Sandy for the misunderstanding. He does some research about transgender cultures and issues and gets advice from a nurse who has a transgender family member. He learns that it is culturally appropriate to refer to transgender individuals as their self-identified gender, regardless of their appearance or level of transition. Ricky recognizes that he made several assumptions about Mrs. Santos and her husband because he was judging them by typical Latino cultural values and comparing Mrs. Santos to the expected prototype of a Latina, perhaps learned in his personal life and reinforced in the cultural competency course. From this experience, you and Ricky realize that true cultural competence is achieved only when clinicians are comfortable with not knowing and not assuming.

### Clinical Pearl

Knowing as much as possible about the cultural background of the communities we serve is definitely valuable, but it is not necessarily useful without a simultaneous process of self-reflection and commitment to lifelong learning in which providers become comfortable letting go of the false sense of security that stereotyping brings. This process mediates enough flexibility and humbleness for providers to recognize when they do not know or understand their patient's belief system. The skill of recognizing this using humility as an approach or philosophy, instead of as a mastered subject or topic, and searching for resources that might enhance the care of the patient and the future practice of the provider are the pillars of cultural humility.

Your assessment reveals that Mrs. Santos is experiencing symptoms that are common when going through the loss of a newborn. You offer her a referral to a grief counselor. You also recommend couples therapy for her and Sandy. You discuss the case with the unit social worker to ensure that Mrs. Santos and Sandy are referred to outpatient therapists who accept their insurance and are welcoming to transgender individuals.

As highlighted previously, this case is incomplete without a description of your own cultural background, traditions, and perceptions and how they relate to Mrs. Santos' symptoms, beliefs, the context in which you relate to her, and the team within which you are providing care.

## DISCUSSION

### Background

The United States has a steadily increasing number of racial and ethnic minorities of varied cultural and linguistic backgrounds. The Census Bureau projects that by 2044, more than half of all Americans will belong to a minority group (Colby & Ortman, 2014). Failing to understand and address social and cultural differences may have significant health consequences for minority groups in particular (Betancourt, Green, Carrillo, & Park, 2002). Academic institutions, accrediting organizations, health care policymakers, and governmental agencies have implemented "cultural competence" as a strategy to improve quality of care for diverse populations and address health equity (Betancourt, Green, Carrillo, & Park, 2005). Several studies support the notion that providing culturally competent services can improve the health of minorities by improving physician–patient communication and delivering health care in the context of each patient's cultural beliefs (Hunt, 2001; Saha, Beach, & Cooper, 2008; Shaya & Gbarayor, 2006). However, sometimes the task of developing cultural competence becomes a vaguely defined goal with very little room for explicit criteria to define its accomplishment (Hunt, 2001), not only because "culture" is a complex and elusive concept but also because "competence" in addressing health disparities requires actions, not just from individual health care providers but also from the whole system.

## Bridging Perspectives and Redefining Concepts

*Culture* has been defined as an integrated pattern of learned core values, beliefs, norms, behaviors, and customs that are shared by a specific group of people (Ring, 2008). It shapes how people perceive reality, acquire a sense of self, think, feel, behave, understand others, and assign meaning to things and events. It can imply a sense of familiarity with others based on perceived similarities or a sense of distance based on perceived differences. Betancourt, Green and Carrillo (2002) define *cultural competence* as the ability of health care systems to provide care to patients with diverse values, beliefs, and behaviors, including tailoring delivery to meet patients' social, cultural, and linguistic needs. This can be a difficult task for systems to achieve.

Cultural competence training often includes courses about normative or traditional values and practices of racial and ethnic minorities. Although this type of training can certainly help providers recognize cultural variants as factors that influence the etiology of health disparities, it bears the risk of training providers to follow "laundry lists of traditional beliefs and practices ostensibly characteristic of particular ethnic groups" (Hunt, 2001, p. 134) and shifts the providers' focus onto how the patient or community differs from their own traditions or from mainstream beliefs, perhaps fostering a sense of disengagement in which mainstream or conventional beliefs become the norm while the "other" becomes the exotic or abnormal.

In order to avoid a rigid or biased kind of cultural competence, providers must understand that "culture" does not imply a blueprint, fixed identity, or body of discrete traits. Instead, it encompasses an ever-changing system of multiple perceptions and actions that individuals can choose from, shaped by the specific socioeconomic context in which it is generated. It is not possible to predict the beliefs and behaviors of individuals based on their cultural background (Hunt, 2001). If providers and health care systems are trained to understand this and to practice with a sense of humility, cultural competence can be taught as a practice principle rather than a false sense of achieved mastery.

## Defining Cultural Humility

The principles of cultural humility first defined by Tervalon and Murray-García (1998) include the following:

- Critical self-reflection: This principle involves full engagement in self-evaluation; acknowledgment of personal assumptions and beliefs; thinking about personal multidimensional cultural identities; and examining personal tendencies toward stigma and discrimination, such as unintentional racism, classism, sexism, ageism, and homophobia.

- Lifelong learning using patient-focused care: Providers use patient-focused interviewing to continuously learn from patients, who are the experts on their own cultures and health beliefs, and even more so on their own needs, goals, and values.
- Recognizing and challenging power imbalances for respectful partnerships: Providers implement the principles described to address provider–patient power imbalances. Collaborative partnerships are developed and maintained not only with patients but also within communities and systems.
- Institutional accountability: Organizations model these principles and undergo a continuous improvement process in order to foster culturally humble practices.

## Cultural Humility and the Social Determinants of Health

Under the social determinants approach, health is not viewed as a distinct entity solely defined as absence of disease or defect but, rather, as interconnected with, and interdependent on, larger systems such as the family, the community, and the environment. Illnesses are defined not only by their pathology but also as the result of imbalances in these systems. Treatments attempt to restore health through analysis of the disturbances in these systems and the restoration of the balance inherent to them. Culture has also been identified as a social determinant of health because it dictates the language used to define issues, the identification and framing of problems, the manner in which solutions are sought, and the methods for defining and measuring success (Knibb-Lamouche, 2012). Providers can use the principles of cultural humility as a framework to become structurally competent in recognizing how social and economic determinants, biases, inequities, and blind spots shape health and illness before and after a clinical encounter (Metzl and Hansen, 2014).

Institutional accountability, in particular, ensures a process in which organizations can identify societal attitudes and policies that might influence the health and health care of disadvantaged patients and communities. In a study analyzing 100 case reports in which a cultural consultation model based on DSM-IV cultural formulation was utilized, the cases demonstrated the impact of cultural misunderstandings: incomplete assessments, incorrect diagnoses, inadequate or inappropriate treatments, and failed treatment alliances (Kirmayer, Groleau, Guzder, Blake, & Jarvis, 2003). By providing cultural humility training and addressing such cultural misunderstandings, organizations can reduce health disparities.

## Implementing Cultural Humility into Systems-Based Practices

The Substance Abuse and Mental Health Services Administration (SAMHSA, 2014) has summarized guidelines for administrators to follow when creating an institutional framework for culturally responsive care delivery, development of policies and procedures, and administrative practices. Most of them are based on the Culturally and Linguistically Appropriate Services (CLAS) standards of the US Department of Health and Human Services, Office of Minority Health (2013). SAMHSA also references requirements for organizational cultural competence, such as defining values and principles, along with demonstrated behaviors, attitudes, policies, and structures that enable effective work across cultures; valuing diversity; conducting self-assessments; managing the dynamics of difference; acquiring and institutionalizing cultural knowledge; and adapting to diversity and the cultural contexts of the communities that organizations serve. Kondrat, Greene, and Winbush (2002) identified the following characteristics of better performing culturally competent organizations: a pro-agency attitude among staff; openness and flexibility of provision; consistent, pro-active, and supportive supervision; and team-based functioning and decision-making.

Utilizing cultural humility principles as the foundation to implement such guidelines can help incorporate systemic practices that truly address health disparities successfully. Self-reflection and institutional accountability can be achieved at the organizational level by incorporating patient satisfaction surveys into assessment processes and providing feedback to clinicians and staff. An example of such surveys is the Iowa Cultural Understanding Assessment–Client Form, adapted from the Assessment Tool for Cultural Competence developed by the Maryland Mental Hygiene Administration of Maryland Health Partners (SAMHSA, 2014; White, Clayton, and Arndt, 2009).

Regarding the concept of humility, a recent study evaluating two hundred and ninety-seven primary care physician–patient interactions demonstrated a relationship between the humility of physicians and the quality of their communication with their patients (Ruberton et al., 2016). This study is believed to be the first empirical research studying this relationship. It concludes that "humble, rather than paternalistic or arrogant, physicians are most effective at working with their patients."

Going beyond competence and utilizing the principles of cultural humility illustrated in this chapter can make a difference in the value that culturally responsive organizational practices can bring to quality in patient outcomes. Furthermore, recognizing power imbalance can promote collaborative partnerships, not only with individual patients, but also within communities and systems.

## REFERENCES

American Psychiatric Association. (2013). Cultural formulation. In *Diagnostic and statistical manual of mental disorders* (5th ed., pp. 749–759). Arlington, VA: American Psychiatric Publishing.

Betancourt, J., Green, A. R., Carrillo, J. E., & Park, E. R. (2002). Cultural competence in Health Care: Emerging Frameworks and Practical Approaches. *The Commonwealth Fund*.

Betancourt, J., Green, A. R., Carrillo, J. E., & Park, E. R. (2005). Cultural competence and health care disparities: Key perspectives and trends. *Health Affairs, 24*(2), 499–505.

Colby, S. L., & Ortman, J. M. (2014). Projections of the size and composition of the US population: 2014 to 2060. *Current Population Reports*, No. 25–1143.Washington, DC: US Census Bureau.

Hunt, L. M. (2001). Beyond cultural competence: Applying humility to clinical settings. *The Park Ridge Center Bulletin, 24*, 3–4. Retrieved from https://www.med.unc.edu/pedclerk/files/hunthumility.pdf

Kirmayer, L. J., Groleau, D., Guzder, J., Blake, C., & Jarvis, E. (2003). Cultural consultation: A model of mental health service for multicultural societies. *Canadian Journal of Psychiatry, 48*, 145–153. Retrieved from https://ww1.cpa-apc.org/Publications/Archives/CJP/2003/april/kirkmayer.pdf

Knibb-Lamouche, J. (2012) Culture as a Social Determinant of Health: Examples from Native Communities. Commissioned paper prepared for the Institute on Medicine, *Roundtable on the Promotion of Health Equity and the Elimination of Health Disparities*. Retrieved from http://nationalacademies.org/hmd/~/media/files/activity%20files/selectpops/healthdisparities/discussion%20and%20commissioned%20papers/culture%20as%20a%20social%20determinant%20of%20health.pdf

Kondrat, M. E., Greene, G., & Winbush, G. (2002). Using benchmarking research to locate agency best practices for African American clients. *Administration and Policy in Mental Health, 29*(6), 495–518.

Metzl, J. M., & Hansen, H. (2014). Structural competency: Theorizing a new medical engagement with stigma and inequality. *Social Science & Medicine, 103*, 126–133.

Ring, J. M. (2008). *Curriculum for culturally responsive health care: The step-by-step guide for cultural competence training*. London, UK: Radcliffe.

Ruberton, P. M., Huynh, H., Miller, T., Kruse, E., Chancellor, J., & Lyubomirsky, S. (2016). The relationship between physician humility, physician–patient communication, and patient health. *Patient Education and Counseling, 99*(7), 1138–1145.

Saha, S., Beach, M. C., & Cooper, L. A. (2008). Patient centeredness, cultural competence and healthcare quality. *Journal of the National Medical Association, 100*(11), 1275–1285.

Shaya, F. T., & Gbarayor, C. M. (2006). The case for cultural competence in health professions education. *American Journal of Pharmaceutical Education, 70*(6), 124.

Substance Abuse and Mental Health Services Administration. (2014). Pursuing organizational cultural competence. In *Improving cultural competence* (Treatment Improvement Protocol (TIP) Series No. 59, pp. 76–96, 273–275). Rockville, MD: Author. Retrieved from https://www.ncbi.nlm.nih.gov/books/NBK248428/pdf/Bookshelf_NBK248428.pdf

Substance Abuse and Mental Health Services Administration. (2014). Appendix C- — Tools for Assessing Cultural Competence: Iowa Cultural Understanding Assessment–Client Form. In *Improving Cultural Competence*. Treatment Improvement Protocol (TIP) Series No. 59, pp. 273–275). Rockville, MD: Author. Retrieved from https://www.ncbi.nlm.nih.gov/books/NBK248429/bin/appc-fm5.pdf

Tervalon, M., & Murray-García, J. (1998). Cultural humility versus cultural competence: A critical distinction in defining physician training outcomes in multicultural education. *Journal of Health Care for the Poor and Underserved, 9*(2), 117–125.

US Department of Health and Human Services, Office of Minority Health. (2013). *National standards for culturally and linguistically appropriate services in health and health care*. Retrieved from https://www.thinkculturalhealth.hhs.gov/assets/pdfs/EnhancedNationalCLASStandards.pdf

White, K., Clayton, R., & Arndt, S. (2009). Culturally Competent Substance Abuse Treatment Project: Annual Report. Iowa Department of Public Health (Contract # 5888CP43). Iowa City, IA: Iowa Consortium for Substance Abuse Research and Evaluation.

# 5

# Harm Reduction

**SONAL BATRA, NOAH VILLEGAS, AND ERIN ZERBO** ■

## CASE HISTORY

Ms. Jacobs is a 32-year-old female with a history of schizoaffective disorder, with one prior hospitalization during a manic episode. At her initial appointment at the community mental health clinic where you work, it appeared that Ms. Jacobs was reluctant to fully disclose details about her life. She presented with heavy make-up and styled hair, but she appeared tired and slightly disheveled. She had erythematous marks on her inner arms that seemed to be recent track marks. Upon discussion, she admitted to using 10 bags of heroin intravenously per day and denied other drug use. She smelled of cigarettes when she came into the office, and she reported smoking one pack of cigarettes per day. She mentioned that she sometimes heard "voices," but she mostly tried to block them out and was not too concerned about them. Her main reason for coming was that she heard this clinic "does Suboxone," and she wanted to try it in order to stop using heroin. She was much more guarded when asked about how she supported herself and who she lived with at home, stating "I get by" and "I have a boyfriend . . . he's ok, it's not too bad." While continuing to obtain history, you start to help her identify treatment goals, with a harm reduction approach in mind.

### Clinical Pearl

*Harm reduction* is defined as a set of policies, programs, and practices aimed at reducing the negative health, social, and economic consequences associated with various behaviors (International Harm Reduction Association, 2010). Classically, it referred to substance use, but its scope has broadened over time to include high-risk sexual activity, nonadherence to treatment, and other behaviors that may lead to negative consequences. While taking a morally neutral and nonjudgmental view, harm reductionists seek to identify specific harms associated with a particular behavior and to develop evidence-based and realistic interventions to reduce those harms. At the same time, a humanistic approach recognizes the dignity and rights of the client, including the right to protection from persecution by the community and the state (Stimson, 2007).

Although harm reduction policies have existed for well over a century, the 1980s saw a more widespread adoption throughout the world as a response to the threat of HIV/AIDS spreading among intravenous drug users. The potential harms of injection opioid use include transmission of HIV and hepatitis B and C, sexually transmitted diseases, overdose, and death. Harm reduction approaches to opioid use include drug substitution for less harmful substances, treatment for opioid cravings, needle exchange programs, providing bleach kits for disinfecting injection equipment, supervised drug injection sites/drug consumption rooms, education and outreach, and increasing access to addiction treatment services. In some places, provision of oral or injectable heroin is even used for harm reduction.

You discuss with Ms. Jacobs the possibility of trying an opioid agonist to treat her heroin use disorder. She was given the option of referral to a nearby methadone clinic, but she preferred a trial of buprenorphine/naloxone. After some education and instructions, she was given a home induction schedule beginning with 8–12 mg on the first day and increasing to 16 mg per day as a maintenance dose. She was referred to the clinic nurse to receive a brief training and prescription for a naloxone take-home kit, which can be used in case of an opioid overdose.

### Clinical Pearl

Medication-assisted treatment (MAT) is the gold standard for opioid use disorders and consists of buprenorphine, methadone, and naltrexone. Buprenorphine and methadone are opioid substitution treatment, and there is strong evidence that their use results in decreased rates of HIV/hepatitis C virus infection, unemployment, crime, and overdose death (Gowing, Farrell, Bornemann, Sullivan, & Ali, 2008). Physicians must complete a training course and obtain a license designation in order to prescribe buprenorphine, a partial opioid agonist. The oral formulations branded Suboxone and Zubsolv contain the combination of buprenorphine/naloxone, which helps prevent intravenous diversion because naloxone is fully bioavailable when injected and will block the "high" but is not absorbed via mucosa, thus rendering it inactive when taken orally as prescribed. Buprenorphine alone (without naloxone) is used for pregnant women and the rare patient with an allergy to naloxone. Methadone has been available since the 1960s via federally regulated "methadone clinics." Patients usually present to the clinic 6 days per week in the beginning and receive a "take-home" dose on Sunday; if urine toxicologies indicate abstinence from substances of abuse, the number of take-home doses can be gradually increased. Usual maintenance doses range from 60 to 120 mg daily, with higher doses correlated with decreased illicit opioid use (American Society of Addiction Medicine, 2015).

Naltrexone (Vivitrol) is the third MAT option, and as an opioid antagonist, it prevents intoxication and also seems to reduce opioid cravings at baseline (Krupitsky et al., 2011). Its use as a monthly injection has been associated with greater retention in treatment, lower relapse rates, and decreased opioid overdose (Lee et al., 2016).

Some researchers have noted a cultural and socioeconomic disparity, with methadone more often the only choice for lower income patients of ethnic minorities (Hansen et al., 2013). There is no evidence to support a difference in effectiveness to explain this disparity, and it is crucial for clinics in the public sector to provide all three options to patients.

Naloxone take-home kits, which contain naloxone vials and syringes or intranasal atomizers, are an effective and low-cost public health intervention to decrease opioid overdose deaths in the community (Breedvelt, Tracy, Dickenson, & Dean, 2015). Kits can be provided to friends and family members who may be the ones to administer the naloxone.

The discussion then turned to Ms. Jacobs' cigarette smoking. She was much more reluctant to address this, stating that "It helps me calm down" and "I just don't feel ready to quit right now." She did note that she had been buying electronic cigarettes on occasion, so she believed she was "already making a change for the better."

### Clinical Pearl

The best option to decrease the burden of disease for smokers is to stop smoking, but for many patients, smoking cessation seems like an insurmountable task. In this instance, the harm reduction approach may be beneficial. Pharmacotherapy (bupropion and varenicline) and nicotine replacement therapy (gum, lozenge, patch, nasal spray, and oral inhaler) can help reduce or replace cigarette use. Relatively recently, the more controversial options, electronic cigarettes and snus, have helped people quit smoking, but they may carry health risks of their own (NIH, 2015; US FDA, 2010). It is unclear if components of the vapor from electronic cigarettes may be carcinogenic (Grana, Benowitz, & Glantz, 2014; Polosa, 2015). The overall cancer-causing risks appear to be lower for the Swedish ingestible moist-tobacco product snus than for smoking, and in one study, 88% of smokers who started using snus stopped smoking (Riley & Pates, 2012; Twombly, 2010). The use of low-nicotine cigarettes, on the other hand, has shown no difference or an increase in cancer risk because people tend to inhale more deeply and smoke more frequently with these "light" cigarettes (Shields, 2002).

After some discussion about the possible risks of electronic cigarettes and education about other smoking cessation methods, Ms. Jacobs ultimately decided that she wanted to defer this issue for the time being.

During the next several sessions, Ms. Jacobs was successfully inducted onto Suboxone and her urine toxicologies indicated she had stopped using heroin. She began attending a few local Narcotics Anonymous meetings, and she agreed to a referral to a substance-focused intensive outpatient program in a nearby hospital to provide her with additional support. Although she admitted to relapsing on intravenous heroin occasionally, often in the context of spending time with friends, she would quickly resume Suboxone afterward and remained motivated to be sober. She reassured you that when she relapsed, she was sure to use clean needles, as you had suggested to her at her first visit.

As time passed, she began to open up more. She revealed that she engaged in sex work in order to support herself and that her boyfriend had introduced her to the "lifestyle" himself and sometimes acted as her "pimp." He was verbally and physically abusive at times, although she remained vague regarding the details and did not express any interest in leaving him.

While taking a supportive approach, you expressed concern regarding Ms. Jacobs's safety. She revealed that although she previously solicited clients on the streets, more recently she had been working out of a "massage parlor," and she believed this was safer. She reported often insisting on the use of condoms with her clients, and she was concerned about the possibility of having a sexually transmitted infection (STI). After providing her STI prevention information, she accepted a referral to a local community health clinic for further testing. While exploring her thoughts on pursuing other avenues of income, she stated, "I want to, but it's not so simple." She also accepted a referral to a local nonprofit organization focused on connecting women with community resources. Although she was reluctant to share specific details about the abuse by her boyfriend, she did seem to be more trusting of you and agreed to create a safety plan for certain situations in which she felt threatened.

### Clinical Pearl

Female sex workers (FSW) often have a history of physical, sexual, and emotional abuse and are at high risk of further abuse (Abad et al., 2015). This may be in the form of abusive clients, abusive intimate partner relationships, or even aggressive law enforcement practices in countries in which sex work remains criminalized. In the United States, with the exception of a few jurisdictions in the state of Nevada, sex work remains illegal. Often, the criminalization and stigmatization of the FSW lifestyle serves to not only marginalize them but also plays a major role in preventing health and education services from reaching them (Riley & Pates, 2012).

Female sex workers are known to be at markedly increased risk of both acquiring and transmitting HIV and other STIs due to involvement in high-risk behaviors. These behaviors may be both voluntary and coerced and include inconsistent use of condoms; sex with multiple partners who themselves are at high risk; and use of multiple substances, including intravenous drug use (Abad et al., 2015; Riley & Pates, 2012).

Significant improvements in the working conditions and support systems of FSW have occurred in countries in which prostitution has been decriminalized. In such locales, harm reduction methods have included free distribution of condoms and training in negotiating condom use with clients; peer education; safety tips and alerts for street-based sex workers; enforcement of occupational health and safety guidelines for brothels; self-help organizations; and offering medical services geared to the needs of FSW, including HIV pre-exposure prophylaxis (Riley & Pates, 2012).

Although it had been deferred, you believed it was important to also address Ms. Jacobs' auditory hallucinations. She quickly became irritable, stating that she would not take any medications because she did not believe they helped and instead made her "fat and sleepy, and like a zombie." She remained insistent that the auditory hallucinations only bothered her when she was stressed, and she re-emphasized that she was able to ignore the voices most of the time.

After determining that there were no imminent safety risks and that Ms. Jacobs remained resolute in her desire to not take medication despite motivational interviewing techniques, a plan was made in collaboration with Ms. Jacobs that included frequent follow-up for monitoring. Stress reduction techniques and specific coping strategies that Ms. Jacobs could use when distressed were also discussed on an ongoing basis. A plan was made to explore possible changes in her attitude toward taking medication in the future.

**Clinical Pearl**

Nonadherence to medications is a common occurrence, and it is a source of frustration for many treatment providers. Some methods to improve adherence have been shown to be effective, such as motivational interviewing, concrete problem-solving, and referral to supportive community services that can help address underlying barriers to adherence. Psychoeducation alone has not been shown to improve adherence (Zygmunt, Olfson, Boyer, & Mechanic, 2002). A clinician may determine that the realities of a particular patient's situation make it more feasible to minimize harms stemming from nonadherence than it may be to eliminate nonadherence (Aldridge, 2012). In such a situation, an alternative approach can incorporate principles of harm reduction. The purpose of such an approach would be to identify, measure, and assess the potential harms related to nonadherence while at the same time balancing the costs and benefits in trying to reduce the harms (Aldridge, 2012). This may include encouraging a gradual rather than an abrupt discontinuation of medication, providing adequate support and ongoing risk assessment, offering psychotherapeutic interventions to manage stress, and reassessing changes in attitude toward medication (Aldridge, 2012).

## DISCUSSION

Countries such as the United Kingdom, the Netherlands, and Australia were early adopters of harm reduction policies (Riley & Pates, 2012). For example, in the mid-1980s, following successes at the local level, the United Kingdom more widely implemented a harm reduction program that included needle exchange, methadone maintenance, outreach and education, and improved access to health care (Stimson, 2007). Officials developed a policy of non-prosecution of individuals found to be in possession of certain types of drug paraphernalia (Riley & Pates, 2012). Throughout the decades, programs have expanded to include other psychoactive substances, and goals have expanded to include reducing the potential harm from overdose as well as from contamination from drugs and drug paraphernalia, reducing exposure of other individuals to drug by-products, and reduction in operation of heavy machinery such as motor vehicles while under the influence.

In the United States, drug policy has continued to be a contentious matter, with prohibition being the primary theme and greatly outweighing promotion of harm reduction. The Harrison Narcotic Act of 1914 criminalized the use of narcotics for treatment of opioid addiction, resulting in the closure of narcotics maintenance clinics (Riley & Pates, 2012). Although methadone maintenance became a major public health initiative starting in the early 1970s (Substance Abuse and Mental Health Services Administration, 2005), the extraordinarily restrictive regulations have had the effect of limiting access to treatment (Novick, Salsitz, Joseph, & Kreek, 2015). Legislation created in the late 1970s criminalized possession of certain drug paraphernalia, such as needles, and this policy was re-emphasized in the late 1980s when legislation aimed at reducing the threat of the AIDS epidemic specifically excluded their provision as a means of harm reduction (Riley & Pates, 2012).

The United States has not conformed with harm reduction policies promoted by a number of United Nations partner organizations and accepted by countries in all regions of the world (Stimson, 2007). As recently as 2011, the US Congress reinstated a ban on federal funding of needle exchange programs (Barr, 2011). By necessity, many of the harm reduction programs in place today have found their leadership and funding from not-for-profit groups and local governments. On a more positive note, the advent of drug court models has helped to usher in a movement toward a more rational and medicalized approach to drug use, which favors treatment over automatic incarceration.

Harm reduction policies continue to be controversial, with opponents citing the danger of failing to suppress harmful behaviors. For example, in the recent past, it was common for many psychiatrists to object to prescribing psychotropic medications to people who were actively using alcohol or drugs, on the grounds that there could be potentially dangerous drug interactions. Some mental health clinics would not treat people with substance use disorders, instead insisting that these people would be better served by a substance abuse program and should return for treatment when sober. However, most psychiatrists now recognize that the benefits of concurrent medication treatment may outweigh the risks and that such treatment may in fact be necessary to help someone with mental illness stop using substances. Another common and challenging example of harm reduction is the prescription of benzodiazepines to people who are dependent on them, tapering slowly to avoid withdrawal symptoms including seizures. These do not seem like harm reduction policies now that they are common practice, but they once were "cutting edge," as other policies may seem to be at this time.

With a patient such as Ms. Jacobs, it is crucial to employ harm reduction strategies to maintain engagement in treatment and achieve the best interim outcomes while still ultimately pursuing long-term recovery goals. It is important to "meet her where she is at," in accordance with patient-centered techniques discussed throughout this book.

## REFERENCES

Abad, N., Baack, B., O'Leary, A., Mizuno, Y., Herbst, J., & Lyles, C. (2015). A systematic review of HIV and STI behavior change interventions for female sex workers in the United States. *AIDS & Behavior, 19*, 1701–1719. doi:10.1007/s10461-015-1013-2

Aldridge, M. A. (2012). Addressing non-adherence to antipsychotic medication: A harm-reduction approach. *Journal of Psychiatric & Mental Health Nursing, 19*, 85–96. doi:10.1111/j.1365-2850.2011.01809.x

American Society of Addiction Medicine. (2015). *The ASAM national practice guideline for the use of medications in the treatment of addiction involving opioid use.* Retrieved from https://www.asam.org/docs/default-source/practice-support/guidelines-and-consensus-docs/asam-national-practice-guideline-supplement.pdf.

Barr, S. (2011, December 21). Needle-exchange programs face new federal funding ban. *Kaiser Health News.* Retrieved from http://khn.org/news/needle-exchange-federal-funding

Breedvelt, J. F., Tracy, D. K., Dickenson, E. C., & Dean, L. V. (2015). "Take home" naloxone: What does the evidence base tell us? *Drugs and Alcohol Today, 15,* 67–75.

Gowing, L., Farrell, M., Bornemann, R., Sullivan, L. E., & Ali, R. (2008). Substitution treatment of injecting opioid users for prevention of HIV infection. *Cochrane Database of Systematic Reviews, 2008*(2), CD004145.

Grana, R., Benowitz, N., & Glantz, S. (2014). E-cigarettes: A scientific review. *Circulation, 129,* 1972–1986. doi:10.1161/circulationaha.114.007667

Hansen, H. B., Siegel, C. E., Case, B. G., Bertollo, D. N., DiRocco, D., Galanter, M. (2013). Variation in use of buprenorphine and methadone treatment by racial, ethnic, and income characteristics of residential social areas in New York City. *Journal of Behavioral Health Services & Research, 40,* 367–377.

Krupitsky, E., Nunes, E.V., Ling, W., Illeperuma, A., Gastfriend, D. R., & Silverman, B. L. (2011). Injective extended-release naltrexone for opioid dependence: A double-blind, placebo-controlled, multicenter randomised trial. *Lancet, 377,* 1506–1513.

Lee, J. D., Friedmann, P. D., Kinlock, T. W., Nunes, E. V., Boney, T. Y., Hoskinson, R. A., Jr., . . . O'Brien, C. P. (2016). Extended-release naltrexone to prevent opioid relapse in criminal justice offenders. *New England Journal of Medicine, 374,* 1232–1242.

National Institutes of Health, National Institute on Drug Abuse. (2015). *Drug facts: Electronic cigarettes (E-cigarettes).* Retrieved from https://www.drugabuse.gov/publications/drugfacts/electronic-cigarettes-e-cigarettes

Novick, D. M., Salsitz, E. A., Joseph, H., & Kreek, M. J. (2015). Methadone medical maintenance: An early 21st-century perspective. *Journal of Addictive Diseases, 34,* 226–237. doi:10.1080/10550887.2015.1059225

Polosa, R. (2015). Electronic cigarette use and harm reversal: Emerging evidence in the lung. *BMC Medicine, 13,* 1–4. doi:10.1186/s12916-015-0298-3

Riley, D. M., & Pates, R. (2012). *Harm reduction in substance use and high-risk behaviour: International policy and practice.* Chichester, UK: Wiley-Blackwell.

Shields, P. (2002). Tobacco smoking, harm reduction, and biomarkers. *Journal of the National Cancer Institute, 94,* 1435–1444. doi:10.1093/jnci/94.19.1435

Stimson, G. (2007). "Harm reduction—Coming of age": A local movement with global impact. *International Journal of Drug Policy, 18,* 67–69.

Substance Abuse and Mental Health Services Administration, Center for Substance Abuse Treatment. (2005). *Medication-assisted treatment for opioid addiction in opioid treatment programs* (Treatment Improvement Protocol (TIP) Series No. 43, pp. 11–24). Retrieved from http://store.samhsa.gov/shin/content/SMA12-4214/SMA12-4214.pdf

Twombly, R. (2010). Snus use in the U.S.: Reducing harm or creating it? *Journal of the National Cancer Institute, 102,* 1454–1456. doi:10.1093/jnci/djq404

US Food and Drug Administration. (2010, September). *E-cigarettes.* Retrieved from https://www.fda.gov

Zygmunt, A., Olfson, M., Boyer, C., & Mechanic, D. (2002). Interventions to improve medication adherence in schizophrenia. *American Journal of Psychiatry, 159,* 1653–1664.

# 6

# Navigating Systems

**S T E P H A N I E   L E   M E L L E**  ■

## CASE HISTORY

Mary is a 52-year-old woman who was diagnosed with schizophrenia at age 24. She receives social security income and lives in her own apartment. Her symptoms usually respond well to a combination of quetiapine and haloperidol, but she has had significant side effects, including insulin intolerance, an 80-pound weight gain, and anticholinergic effects. Now Mary presents with worsening symptoms attributable to decreased adherence to medications. She states, "I get confused about which pill to take." She is followed in a medical clinic for insulin-dependent diabetes. The primary care provider (PCP) at this clinic is frustrated with her nonadherence with medical care. Mary also has difficulty sticking to her diet and spends most of her time in her apartment because she is afraid of "bad people" in her neighborhood and is tired all the time.

### Clinical Pearl

#### Complicated Lives—Multiple Systems of Care

Many people whom we serve in public-sector behavioral health have more than just their mental illness with which to contend. We use the term "social determinants of health" to describe and evaluate other aspects of peoples' lives that contribute to their ability to maintain wellness. These include social, economic, and environmental circumstances, in addition to gender, age, and race/ethnicity (World Health Organization and Calouste Gulbenkian Foundation, 2014). To provide effective mental health treatment for people with serious mental illness and complex needs, we must take a systematic approach—that is, systems-based practices—that starts with an assessment of each system. The assessment may include mental health, substance abuse, physical health, housing, benefits, family/social, vocational/educational, and legal systems (Lemelle, Arbuckle, & Ranz, 2013).

Mary's labs, drawn in your clinic, show that her blood glucose level has been in the 200–300 range. Mary's health may deteriorate if her diabetes is not better controlled. She tells you that she would agree to take insulin but that she cannot afford the co-payment on her medication and medical supplies. You also find out that Mary's sister, who also has mental illness, has moved in with Mary and is financially dependent on her, which is a major stressor for Mary.

### Clinical Pearl

#### Systems-Based Practices (SBP)

The Accreditation Council of General Medical Education (ACGME, 2015) describes SBP as an "awareness of and responsiveness to the larger context and system of health care, as well as the ability to call effectively on other resources in the system to provide optimal health care" (p. 16; see also Swick, Hall, & Beresin, 2006).

Psychiatrists frequently perform SBP, but it is difficult to describe, operationalize, and teach SBP. Ranz et al. (2012) performed a study involving 12 residency programs nationally to determine the components of SBP as taught in psychiatry residency training. The study resulted in the four factor model of SBP, which delineates a set of roles performed by psychiatrists to meet the comprehensive needs of the patient within and beyond the health care system. The roles, described in Box 6.1, are patient care advocate, team member, information integrator, and resource manager. Here, Mary's case is used to examine these four roles of SBP.

In your role as patient care advocate, you engage Mary in a review of all the systems that are affecting her health, including her mental and physical health, finances, social supports, and daily activities. Mary wants to start with her relationship with her sister. She states that she feels responsible for her sister, but she is used to living alone and believes that her sister may be spying on her. You believe that Mary's psychotic and diabetic symptoms may be interfering with her ability to care for herself and to access the additional services she needs. After some discussion, Mary agrees to prioritize her mental and physical health. Mary states, "If I feel better I will be able to deal with my sister better." You and Mary develop a plan to use a pillbox for her medications, and you plan to have a family meeting with her sister.

### Clinical Pearl

#### Patient Care Advocate Role

Central to the role of patient care advocate is the development of a trusting relationship, using shared decision-making and advocating for the person's needs. This includes developing a dynamic understanding of the person as well as a person-centered and recovery-oriented treatment plan for symptom management. This is the role that clinicians most often carry out, and it is taught throughout medical training.

In your role as team member, you realize that you need to involve other members of the multidisciplinary team as well as Mary's sister in her care. You have a family meeting with Mary and her sister, and you find out that her sister is willing to help Mary with household chores and to help Mary stick to her diet. Also, Mary's sister states that she is searching for a job. You contact the clinic nurse and ask her to help Mary learn to fill her pillbox. You also contact Mary's PCP, who states that Mary is often a "no show" and that when she does come in, she will not wait in the waiting

BOX 6.1

**FOUR ROLES OF SYSTEMS-BASED PRACTICES**

*Patient care advocate*: One-on-one relationship with the person, advocating for the person's needs
- Person-centered care: Able to describe care from the person's perspective and convey this to others
- Engagement: Develops a meaningful relationship with the person
- Shared decision-making: Involves the person in planning and carrying out treatment
- Ongoing evaluation and anticipation: Responds to the evolving needs of the person
- Advocacy for patients' needs: Representing patients at the program, local, state, or national level

*Team member*: Working toward a common goal
- Role definition: Describes roles and contribution of team members
- Facilitation: Seeks out team member input and shares it with the rest of the team
- Education: Actively contributes to the team, sharing perspectives and knowledge about the person's clinical and social condition
- Supervision: Organizes team meetings and/or supervises individual team members, negotiating conflicts

*Information integrator*: Gather, analyze, and effect change
- Documentation: Describes the person's clinical symptoms and also describes systems of care based on the person's psychosocial needs
- Data analysis: Aggregates and prioritizes accumulated data from multiple systems
- Treatment planning: Uses available information and literature to develop a best-practice treatment plan
- Systems change: Designs and implements a program evaluation or continuous quality improvement project to improve services

*Resource manager*: Recognize resource needs and match with available resources
- Micro resources: Analyzes the person's financial and social resources, and goods and services available to the patient
- Macro resources: Analyzes the financial and social resources, and goods and services available in the larger system
- The principle of justice: Balances a person's needs with the resources available in a system
- Management decisions: Considers the system-wide distribution of both micro and macro resources
- Policy: Develops policies and procedures based on micro and macro needs on a program, organization, or national level

room. You share information about Mary's new treatment plan with the PCP and arrange for Mary to go to the medical clinic with her sister. You also agree to give each other updates on Mary's progress by e-mail.

### Clinical Pearl

### Team Member

Central to the role of team member is an understanding of the unique expertise that each team member brings to the care of a person. We often need to include team members from outside the traditional multidisciplinary team. Team members can be family or friends, people who work in housing programs or benefits offices, or other clinicians. Anyone who provides care or services for an individual may be recruited as a team member. With the development of collaborative care programs and the increasing need for coordination with managed care organizations (MCOs), our teams have become larger and more complex, but with the addition of each new team member comes the potential for improved coordinated care.

For a team to work effectively, there must be a common goal, and all team members contribute to reaching that goal. The team leader must keep the team on track and must manage conflicting interests between team members and with the person. When goals are not being met, this may be a sign that new or different team members are needed. In Mary's case, involving her sister in addition to engaging her PCP allowed her physical health needs to be better met.

In your role as information integrator, you discuss with Mary's PCP your concerns about her medical care. As a result of the information shared, you realize that Mary will not let her PCP draw her labs. You arrange for Mary's labs drawn in your clinic to be faxed to her PCP, and you also discuss her concerns about having labs drawn at her PCP's office.

You also find out from Mary's sister that the stove in their apartment does not work, so they have been eating fast food daily. To better meet Mary's physical health needs, you share this information with the social worker in your clinic, who is able to contact the landlord about repairing the stove. The nurse also shares information about healthy eating with Mary and her sister.

### Clinical Pearl

### Information Integrator

Central to the role of information integrator is the collection of crucial data from multiple team members and systems. These data must then be analyzed and used to effect change in either a person's treatment plan or in a system of care. The roles of information integrator and team member go hand in hand. Team members are the people representing multiple systems of care from whom we gather data/information. In this case, the information from the PCP resulted in a systems change that affected how Mary's lab results were shared, and the information from Mary's sister resulted in increased services.

Information integration also includes sharing information across larger systems of care, including between health providers and MCOs. New software and health information organizations have been developed to share electronic records between hospital and provider systems for individuals who consent to this. Many of these large information sharing systems also have "patient portals" that allow clients to participate in information integration.

In your role as resource manager, you explore with Mary her financial situation. Mary explains that after paying her rent, she has only approximately $200 left for other expenses. Mary states that she and her sister are eating fast food because that is all that they can afford. Mary also states that her sister is searching for a job now and does not have time to take Mary to her appointments or to the grocery store. Mary is afraid to go out of the house by herself and is feeling more isolated, even with her sister around. Mary asks if there is anyone else who might be able to help her outside of her home. The clinic is currently short staffed, and the case manager who was working with Mary recently retired. All the other case managers are over-worked, so you try to get one of the social work students to help Mary fill her pillbox and take her to appointments and the grocery store. The social work student is new to the area and is not familiar with community resources, but he is willing to learn.

### Clinical Pearl

**Resource Manager**
Central to the resource manager role is management of the person's resource needs and availability (micro resources) and the system's resource needs and availability (macro resources). The actual resources to be managed include financial, human, material, and time resources. This is most challenging when the person's needs cannot be met by the resources available in a system of care. The resource manager role is the one role that we are least trained to perform, and it is often the role that is the most frustrating (Graham et al., 2009; Graham, Naqvi, Encandela, Harding, & Chatterji, 2009).

In this case, Mary has significant needs: (1) financial needs that affect her ability to afford a healthy diet and her co-pay for medications; (2) human needs that affect her ability to navigate the community and fill her pillbox; (3) material needs that affect her access to treatment; and (4) time needs, which include scheduling Mary's time, her sister's time, and the clinical staff time to work with Mary and her other team members.

In this case, the system—Mary's clinic—is lacking in human resources and does not have resources that might enhance access to care, such as a community outreach program or provision of transportation to the clinic. As advocates not only for individual patients but also for a population of patients, public psychiatrists search for creative solutions to system-wide resource shortages. To address micro resource deficiencies in Mary's case, you used a flexible resource, the social work student, to fill a system gap. However, this is not a stable solution. Advocating with clinic or agency management, managed care, or government leaders for adequate service resources can address the macro resource deficiencies in our systems.

## DISCUSSION

The four factor model of SBP is a conceptual framework that operationalizes how we interact with people and systems on a regular basis. This model is helpful when working with people who have complex needs that involve multiple systems of care. You will usually start in the role of patient care advocate, but you might conceptually change roles to that of a resource manager if the patient's concrete needs are impacting his or her health care or to a team member if the patient's current needs require the skill set of one of your colleagues. This model can also be used as a supervisory tool (Le Melle, Clemmey, & Ranz, 2014). It gives us a common language for teaching the complexities of SBP. Psychiatrists' accreditation now requires competency in SBP, and the four factor model was used to inform the milestone requirements for SBP (Widge, Hunt, & Servis, 2014).

The systems in which we provide health care are changing. We are beginning to understand and incorporate social determinants of health in our treatment of the whole person. We now realize that targeting symptom remission is not enough to improve peoples' lives. People with mental illnesses disproportionately experience socioeconomic challenges that, in turn, affect their journeys to recovery. We must consider all the systems that affect health, such as housing, income, employment, and meaningful social activities.

In their roles as patient care advocates, public psychiatrists have led a number of efforts to address system-wide barriers to recovery for people with mental illnesses. A prominent example is the Housing First model, which asserts that people cannot achieve recovery without decent housing (Tsemberis & Eisenberg, 2000). In this model, people with mental illness are given housing as a first treatment step, instead of having to demonstrate psychiatric stability before being housed. Success in ventures such as these brings hope to both patients and providers frustrated by resource scarcities that impact care.

The US public health system has significant challenges in terms of coordination and integration of care, with numerous providers maintaining separate health records and often not communicating with other providers for a given patient. Among systems solutions to these issues are health homes, which have the capacity to provide outreach and coordinate resources in ways that traditional programs cannot. Health home care managers (differently named in different localities) "apply systems, science, incentives, and information to improve medical practice and assist consumers and their support system to become engaged in a collaborative process designed to manage medical/social/mental health conditions more effectively" (Center for Health Care Strategies, 2007, p. 1). In some cases, this work can be supported by MCO efforts to coordinate care, which are motivated both by patient outcomes and by reduction in unnecessary costs related to utilization of emergency or inpatient services. Part of the role of both a team member and a resource manager is to understand how health homes and MCOs work and how to integrate them into the treatment team.

Working with these expanded health care teams requires skill as an information integrator. These expanded teams may be co-located or virtual teams that use electronic and telemedicine technologies to support communication. Health information exchanges also permit data sharing between separate electronic health records, with a patient's consent. One challenge with such information exchanges is that an enormous amount of data may be made available—more than can be reasonably integrated. Data management systems that help us identify useful and important information and stratify risk are in constant development.

Outcomes are perhaps the most important piece of data—one that is monitored by MCOs and other health care payers that use quality, productivity, and other outcome measures as criteria for funding. As resource managers, psychiatrists may thus be involved in monitoring outcomes for their patients and for the systems in which they work. The interesting fact that the aforementioned Housing First model was championed by a conservative federal administration, due to the research evidence for its success, highlights the importance of outcomes monitoring to all four roles of SBP.

Using the four factor model of SBP to inform a systems approach to care allows psychiatrists to broaden their roles beyond simply evaluator and prescriber. We can be skilled managers who provide recovery-oriented, person-centered care in complex systems, and we can be leaders in the changing field of behavioral health.

## REFERENCES

Accreditation Council for Graduate Medical Education. (2015). *ACGME program requirements for graduate medical education in psychiatry: Effective July 1, 2017*. Retrieved from https://www.acgme.org/Portals/0/PFAssets/ProgramRequirements/400_psychiatry_2017-07-01.pdf

Center for Health Care Strategies. (2007). *Care management definition and framework*. Retrieved from http://www.chcs.org/usr_doc/Care_Management_Framework.pdf. Accessed November 15, 2016.

Graham, M. J., Naqvi, Z., Encandela, J. A., Bylund, C. L., Dean, R., Calero-Breckheimer, A., & Schmidt, H. J. (2009). What indicates competency in systems-based practice? An analysis of perspective consistency among healthcare team members. *Advances in Health Sciences Education: Theory and Practice, 14*(2), 187–203.

Graham, M. J., Naqvi, Z., Encandela, J., Harding, K. J., & Chatterji, M. (2009). Systems-based practice defined: Taxonomy development and role identification for competency assessment of residents. *Journal of Graduate Medical Education, 1*(1), 49–60.

Le Melle, S., Arbuckle, M., & Ranz, J. (2013). Integrating systems-based practice, community psychiatry, and recovery into residency training. *Academic Psychiatry, 37*(1), 35–37.

Le Melle, S., Clemmey, P., & Ranz, J. (2014). Outpatient training in public/community psychiatry and systems-based practices. *Academic Psychiatry, 38*(6), 693–695.

Ranz, J., Weinberg, M., Arbuckle, M. R., Fried, J., Carino, A., McQuistion, H. L., . . . Vergare, M. J. (2012). A four factor model of systems-based practices in psychiatry. *Academic Psychiatry, 36*(6), 473–478.

Swick, S., Hall, S., & Beresin, E. (2006). Assessing the ACGME competencies in psychiatry training programs. *Academic Psychiatry, 30*(4), 330–351.

Tsemberis, S., & Eisenberg, R. R. (2000). Pathways to housing: Supported housing for street-dwelling homeless individuals with psychiatric disabilities. *Psychiatric Services, 51*(4), 487–493.

Widge, A., Hunt, J., & Servis, M. (2014). Systems-based practice and practice-based learning for the general psychiatrist: Old competencies, new emphasis. *Academic Psychiatry, 38*(3), 288–293.

World Health Organization and Calouste Gulbenkian Foundation. (2014). *Social determinants of mental health*. Geneva, Switzerland: World Health Organization.

# 7

# Financing Care

A N I T A   E V E R E T T ◾

## CASE HISTORY

Brian Lusby is a 44-year-old man who was found under a bridge and brought to the Your Best Hospital (YBH) emergency department (ED) by the Homeland police behavioral unit. He was sunburned and disheveled. He reported "looking for his people in the promised land," and he refused admission because he did not want to "waste my time or cloud my judgment day." In answer to questions about his most recent meal, he reported "missions, kitchens, health, and death, I went to MIT and I am not coming back."

Brian was evaluated by the YBH psychiatrist on call; Brian was disorganized, psychotic, and unable to make rational decisions regarding his safety. Civil commitment proceedings were initiated. He was asked about his health insurance, and his reply was "Insurance is the devil's work."

Brian was unable to give virtually any details of his life or medical history. Review of the record revealed an admission to YBH 2 years ago, following the death of his mother. He had several outpatient visits in the YBH mental health clinic after the hospitalization. The last outpatient note refers to his brother's insistence that he move to his brother's home in a neighboring state, Newland.

He was uninsured at the last admission, but he was eligible for an uncompensated care program and was able to be seen at the clinic through a city-operated community grant program. A city grant program provided vouchers for medications on a limited formulary for uncompensated care patients, which enabled him to be maintained on haloperidol.

### Clinical Pearl

Persons with serious mental illnesses are much more likely to have government-sponsored insurance, such as Medicaid and Medicare, compared to persons with general medical conditions. Often, state, city, or county government programs are needed to close gaps in services funding. Learning to navigate the health care financing system so that your patient receives needed treatment and rehabilitative services is an essential part of a public psychiatrist's work, and psychiatrists have a valuable role in advocating for better access to care.

Emergency staff are eventually able to reach Brian's brother Gary in Newland, who is extremely relieved that Brian has been found. He relates that Brian had been living with him for several months after their mother had died. Gary explained that Brian was initially doing well. Gary then adds,

> We tried to pay for his treatment, but we just could not keep up. He was doing so well for a while. He helped at home and he came into work with me at my engineering firm 2 days a week. I promised my mother I would look after him. We could manage the cost when he was on Haldol, but the Newland doctor recommended a new medicine because of side effects, and the new medication was several hundred dollars a month. We talked to other families at National Alliance on Mental Illness and we learned that he might be eligible for Medicaid in Newland—this was very hard for us—it was a big relief to find out we might be able to get some help.

Gary further relates,

> With Medicaid in Newland, we were able to get that expensive medication. He had a case manager and he enrolled in a supported employment program. They were going to help him find an apartment. Then things started falling apart. He stayed in his room, and then he refused to go to the program.

Suddenly Brian disappeared, and they had not heard from him in several weeks.

### Clinical Pearl

Brian's family was able to pay for his care initially, until the cost of his treatment became prohibitive. Traditionally, a greater proportion of the total spending for mental health services comes from out-of-pocket payment than is the case for other health services. Many psychiatrists do not participate in Medicaid or Medicare, and some do not participate in any insurance programs. This is often because the reimbursement rates are low and do not reflect the time cost of providing complex psychosocial treatments.

Brian was fortunate in that the Medicaid program in Newland had a wide array of services for beneficiaries with serious mental illness. Eligibility for Medicaid varies from state to state. Medicaid may pay for expanded rehabilitation services, but it cannot be utilized to pay for services that are not medical, such as housing or job placement services. When supported housing or employment coaching is characterized as rehabilitative, components of these services can be paid for by Medicaid. In some states, Medicaid is partnered with services or funding from a state or local government department of housing or human resources to piece together services.

Gary said that Brian had become ill while in his first semester of college at Massachusetts Institute of Technology. He became socially withdrawn, developed paranoid delusions about his physics professor, and was hospitalized. He returned home to live with his parents in Homeland and remained with them until his mother died. Although he was never able to return to college, he was engaged in his community and his life had meaning. He was married briefly and had two serious suicide attempts in the year after the divorce. These suicide attempts were associated with psychiatric hospitalizations, including a 6-month stay at Homeland State Psychiatric Hospital.

### Clinical Pearl

Historically, state hospitals were funded directly from state government funds, and patients were not billed for treatment. A controversial component of Medicaid has been the "IMD exclusion," with IMD standing for Institution for Mental Diseases. An IMD is a freestanding inpatient psychiatric treatment facility with 16 or more beds. State hospitals and many other freestanding psychiatric hospitals that are IMDs cannot bill Medicaid for treatment. This has provided incentives for states to reduce the number of state-funded psychiatric beds and to use Medicaid (matched by federal funds) to provide inpatient treatment in non-IMD psychiatric settings, such as psychiatric units in general hospitals.

In Homeland in the ED, YBH is able to admit Brian to its a 24-bed psychiatric unit. Brian is treated with olanzapine and lorazepam, and after several days he is able to communicate more spontaneously. He reveals that the employment program in Newland was encouraging him to "follow his dreams" to work in an engineering office and he had begun taking some engineering courses. Brian found that he could not focus on the calculus problems, and he stopped taking his medication in order to think more clearly. This was a stressor that he was embarrassed to discuss with his brother. After several weeks, things were not going well and he left his brother's home so that he would not be a burden. By returning to Homeland, he hoped to start over.

After 5 days in the psychiatric unit, Brian is more organized and able to participate in discharge planning. He wants to live in Homeland, where he has lived all his life. However, he is not eligible for Medicaid in Homeland, and the city-funded programs in which he previously participated are no longer in place, so he would not be able to obtain ongoing treatment there. After talking with Gary, he decides to return to Newland.

### Clinical Pearl

If Brian were able to remain longer in the hospital, the inpatient team would have time to resolve some of the health care financing issues that prevent him from remaining in Homeland. It is very common for contemporary psychiatric units to have very short lengths of stay. Historically, psychiatric hospitals were able to work with individuals for months and years; today, there is pressure to manage the costs of inpatient treatment. Often, there is tension between the insurance entity, incentivized to manage costs, and the clinical team, which has a responsibility to ensure that the person is well enough to function safely in the community. Discharge planning is essential so that the ongoing treatment can effectively be managed by a receiving outpatient provider.

In Newland, Gary helps Brian reconnect with his case management agency, which helps Brian find a bed in a group home. He is discouraged that he "failed" in the programs his brother had helped him get into. His mental health team actively works with him to restore hope for recovery. They are reviewing the possibility of him restarting the supported employment program, this time with closer monitoring. At the same time, his case manager suggests that he apply for social security disability (SSD). This will ensure that he receives income and Medicare on an ongoing basis.

### Clinical Pearl

Once approved for SSD, and after a 2-year mandatory waiting period, disabled individuals become Medicare recipients. Unlike Medicaid, Medicare is completely funded and managed by the federal government. Approximately 85% of Medicare recipients are elderly; approximately 15% are adults with disabilities. Individuals may qualify for both Medicare and Medicaid; these individuals may be referred to as "duals." Typically, Medicare has a benefits package that is similar to that of private insurance, covering inpatient, outpatient, and professional fees. Medicare does not cover psychiatric rehabilitation services. Medicaid is the "payer of last resort," covering services that Medicare does not. If Brian becomes a dual, Medicare will become his first payer, and Medicaid will only pay for those services that Medicare does not provide.

## DISCUSSION

Medicaid is the single largest funder of treatment for persons with behavioral health conditions in the United States. Medicaid is a state–federal partnership. States design eligibility and benefits, and these must be in accord with federal Centers for Medicare and Medicaid Services (CMS) rules (https://www.cms.gov). The federal financial contribution to a state's Medicaid program varies by state per capita income and has always been 50% or more of the cost. Medicaid was enacted in 1965 and was originally created to provide insurance for children in poor families so that these children had opportunity to access preventive and sick child services on par with other children. Although Medicaid was originally projected to be a small program for poor children, it has grown considerably and is now the major safety net insurance for Americans with limited financial means. Medicaid provides for many services for adults with serious mental illnesses that are not covered as benefits in Medicare or commercial insurance plans. The Patient Protection and Affordable Care Act of 2010 provided federal funding that was designed to reduce the total number of uninsured adults by raising the Medicaid eligibility income level in states that chose to participate. Ongoing concerns about Medicaid include the typically low rates of reimbursement for services and the fact that much of Medicaid is based on a fee-for-service payment model that incentivizes the number of services provided rather than rewarding improved care quality and health outcomes.

Basic working knowledge about the interrelationship between Medicaid and Medicare is useful in establishing what options a dual patient has for inpatient and outpatient treatment and medication. For example, generally Medicare has broader medication formularies compared to Medicaid managed care programs. However, there are some rehabilitation services that are not covered by Medicare that may be covered by Medicaid. Given that duals are usually disabled adults who are of limited financial means, these patients are at high risk of poor health outcomes and may incur high costs associated with emergency and inpatient service use; they therefore need high-quality, coordinated care.

Typically, access to mental health treatment is more limited than that for medical/surgical care, particularly for people who have commercial insurance plans or who do not have insurance. One factor that resulted in more out-of-pocket payment is the higher co-pays that have historically been charged for behavioral health services. The Mental Health Parity and Addiction Equity Act of 2008 and related state parity laws have theoretically put the management and payment for behavioral health services on more equal footing with all health services.

Much of US health care policy occurs through incremental changes. Historically, there have been several efforts to move toward something like a single-payer system, recognizing the superior health outcomes and lower costs associated with single-payer systems in other countries (Grob & Goldman, 2006). One example of a change effort specific to behavioral health was the passage of President Kennedy's Community Mental Health Act (CMHA) in 1963, which provided grants to states to establish community mental health centers. Only half of the proposed centers were built, and the CMHA did not provide ongoing financial support. The CMHA enabled the deinstitutionalization of people with serious mental illness, but it was unable to provide sufficient community care to receive them (Torrey, 2014).

Recent trends in health care financing include value-based payment. Value ($V$) is equal to the quality ($Q$) of a service divided by the cost to deliver that service ($C$). A simple formula might be $V = Q/C$ so that greater quality with lower cost results in greater value. Recently, there has been increasing attention to the rising costs of health care in the United States without commensurate quality. National health care outcomes including lifespan, infant mortality rates, and other health care indicators in the United States have lagged far behind metrics for other economically advanced countries (World Health Organization, 2016). A fee-for-service system works for well people with single problems that can be addressed in an episode of treatment. However, people with multiple and chronic conditions are often cost drivers and require highly coordinated, prevention-oriented care.

Managed care organizations (MCOs) are charged with reducing the cost of care in order to achieve either a profit margin (for-profit MCOs) or a balanced budget (not-for-profit MCOs), but they must compete to achieve higher health outcomes, both to attract participants to their insurance plans and to meet federal and state regulations governing quality of care. MCOs manage costs by determining basic benefits and by limiting outlier high-cost services such as long lengths of stay and expensive medications. Sometimes, these coverage rules can be barriers to care or cause unnecessary burdens, requiring provider advocacy to shape the patient–provider–payer dynamic. The more responsive MCOs have promoted care quality metrics and care coordination programs as ways of improving quality and reducing costs.

Emerging evidence supports the notion that treating behavioral health conditions helps reduce total health care costs (Kathol, Degruy, & Rollman, 2014).

Increasingly, advocates can educate officials and lawmakers on the value of behavioral health care and rehabilitation programs, including supported housing and employment.

Understanding how services are financed enables psychiatrists and health care providers to better care for patients and to be leaders and advocates for system improvement. The financing "puzzle pieces" come together to provide, at the very least, a safety net and, at optimum, a high-quality delivery system that promotes resilience, recovery, and well-being.

## REFERENCES

Grob, G., & Goldman, H. (2006). *The dilemma of federal mental health policy: Radical reform or incremental change.* Piscataway, NJ: Rutgers University Press.

Kathol, R. G., Degruy, F., & Rollman, B. L. (2014). Value-based financially sustainable behavioral health components in patient centered medical homes. *Annals of Family Medicine, 12*, 172–175.

Torrey, F. (2014). *American psychosis.* New York, NY: Oxford University Press.

World Health Organization. (2016). *World health statistics 2016: Monitoring health for the sustainable development goals.* Geneva, Switzerland: Author.

# Across the Lifespan

# 8

# Early Childhood Mental Health

*Prevention and Intervention*

**J. REBECCA WEIS ■**

## INTRODUCTORY NOTE

Early childhood mental health is inextricably linked to parental mental health, so both are covered in the case presented in this chapter.

## CASE HISTORY

Joyce is a 23-year-old female admitted to labor and delivery. This is her first child, and she is anxious because she has not been able to reach the father of the baby. She received prenatal care at a local clinic and reports "good health," although she admits she was psychiatrically hospitalized 2 years ago. She has no current psychiatric treatment. Delivery proceeds without complications, and when her partner arrives, he seems supportive. As part of a program that the hospital had set up in collaboration with a psychiatrist, Joyce is screened for depression. Her score is mildly elevated, and she tells the social worker that the symptoms identified on the screen have been present for several weeks. The social worker gives her an appointment at the hospital's mental health clinic for 2 weeks after discharge.

### Clinical Pearl

Depression and anxiety disorders affect up to 20% of women during and after pregnancy. Rates may be even higher among mothers with risk factors such as poverty and poor social support. The American College of Obstetrics and Gynecologists (2015) recommends screening all mothers for depression during the perinatal period. Table 8.1 lists two commonly used instruments in the public domain.

Screening using standardized questionnaires improves identification, but obstetric providers may be reluctant to screen without having a plan to deal with positive screens. Psychiatrists sometimes provide support through traditional

*Table 8.1* EXAMPLES OF SCREENING INSTRUMENTS USED IN
THE PUBLIC DOMAIN

| Screening Instrument | Sensitivity | Specificity | No. of Questions | Language Availability |
|---|---|---|---|---|
| EPDS (cut-off score of 13)[a] | 0.63–0.94 | 0.83–0.98 | 10 | >35 languages |
| PHQ-9[b] | 0.75–0.85 | 0.84–0.88 | 9 | >30 languages |

[a]EPDS, Edinburgh Postnatal Depression Scale—also useful during pregnancy (Cox, Holden, & Sagovsky, 1987).
[b]PHQ, Patient Health Questionnaire (Kroenke, Spitzer, & Williams, 2001).

consultative functions in hospital settings, but they will only be able to see a certain percentage of patients. By working on a systemic level to help medical colleagues develop good plans for screening and referrals, the public psychiatrist's reach is expanded.

At baby Susannah's 1-month well-baby visit, Joyce bursts into tears, claiming she is a "terrible mother." The pediatrician becomes worried. He learns Joyce has a history of depression and that she missed her mental health clinic appointment. On a depression screening instrument, she now scores in the moderate depression range. Joyce is willing to get help, but she has felt embarrassed about calling to reschedule her missed appointment. A social worker in the clinic makes the call with her. In addition, the social worker refers Joyce to a program providing home-visiting services to new mothers.

### Clinical Pearl

The American Academy of Pediatrics also recommends maternal depression screening given compelling evidence that addressing maternal depression has a positive impact for children; however, pediatricians also need clearly established pathways to get mothers help. Again, psychiatrists can play a critical role in helping with workflow development. Use of standardized tools to track early childhood social–emotional development is also emerging as a best practice in pediatrics.

To address symptoms when they are found through screening, some pediatric clinics choose to co-locate mental health providers familiar with early childhood and maternal mental health (Olin et al., 2015). The Healthy Steps for Young Children program (Women's and Children's Health Policy Center, 2003) is a flexible model for implementing early childhood collaborative care in pediatric practices.

When maternal mental health services are not readily available in the practice, referral to a mental health clinic will need to be arranged. The pediatric practice will also need to follow up with the mother to ensure that the referral succeeds, because many referrals are not successful the first time.

Telephone consultation models can also be helpful given the overall shortage of mental health services in many communities. For instance, Massachusetts has developed a phone consultation model staffed by psychiatrists to assist primary care providers (MCPAP for Moms, n.d.).

Home visiting programs such as the Nurse Family Partnership (Olds et al., 2010) and Healthy Families America (http://www.healthyfamiliesamerica.org) provide support, developmental guidance, and parent coaching. Although not "treatment," home visits are effective and especially useful for families who may have difficulty getting to clinic appointments.

Joyce goes to the appointment and is diagnosed with major depressive disorder. Importantly, the evaluation concludes that there is no acute danger to the baby or the mother. Joyce requests psychotherapy rather than medication because she is still trying to breast-feed.

During the next month, Joyce meets three times with the therapist. She explores her many recent life transitions—starting a new relationship, moving out of her mother's apartment and into her partner's, learning that her partner had a significant psychiatric history, and becoming a mother. She also talks about her goals as a mother. She comes to understand that all the recent transitions and the isolation she feels being home so much with the baby contribute to her depressed mood. She formulates short-term goals to get outside at least briefly each day and to reconnect with a friend. She learns relaxation strategies to use when stressed. She reports a significant decrease in symptoms on the Edinburgh Postnatal Depression Scale (EPDS) and is clearly more interactive with Susannah, who responds in kind with bright and engaging smiles for her mother.

### Clinical Pearl

Perinatal depression has the potential to interfere with mother–infant interactions. Infant development and attachment are supported by "mother's use of positive affect, infant-directed speech, affectionate touch, and maternal responsiveness" (Lefkovics, Baji, & Rigo, 2014). As maternal depression symptoms improve, clinicians will also often observe positive changes in the dyadic relationship.

Joyce does not return for the next therapy appointment. The therapist calls her and learns she has returned to work; thus, she cannot meet weekly. Joyce also mentions that she is pregnant. The therapist suggests prenatal care at the hospital clinic so they can check in during her OB appointments. The pregnancy is uneventful for the first trimester, but then Joyce's partner stops taking his medication, develops paranoia, and accuses her of having an affair. One evening, he strikes her on the face. Joyce takes Susannah to her mother's apartment. She learns a few days later that her partner left the country. Joyce moves in with her mother because she cannot afford housing on her own. Fortunately, neither Joyce nor the fetus were injured, but she is distressed both by the recent trauma and by the strain in her relationship with her mother. She meets with her therapist, who suggests meeting more regularly because her EPDS score had increased dramatically. Joyce also meets with the psychiatrist, and he recommends adding an antidepressant.

Joyce's mother helps out with Susannah, but Joyce then feels guilty about not being able to "mother" her daughter. With Joyce's permission, the therapist contacts Joyce's home visitation program. They are able to increase the frequency of home visits to provide extra support for the relationship between Joyce and Susannah.

Joyce's symptoms stabilize. She carries her pregnancy to full-term and delivers a healthy baby boy, Michael. During the next several months, she tapers her therapy and medication.

### Clinical Pearl

Although Joyce initially responded well to psychotherapy, the evolution of new stressors resulted in relapse. The social worker and psychiatrist in this case were able to make rapid clinical adjustments to help Joyce. The impact of antidepressants during pregnancy (and breast-feeding) for child outcomes is a subject of active research; however, given that severe depression and stress also carry risks during and after pregnancy, the benefits of treatment in some cases outweigh potential risks of a medication. Because the literature continues to evolve on this topic, any prescriber working with pregnant women will need to stay abreast of new information.

When Michael turns 3 years old, he starts preschool, where his behavior is difficult to manage. The preschool teacher suggests an evaluation with the Early Childhood Mental Health Consultant who is on-site once per week, but Joyce is initially reluctant, worried that Michael will be labeled a "problem child." She agrees to start with completing an Early Childhood Screening Assessment questionnaire (see Table 8.2). In reviewing her answers, she realizes she is also seeing challenging behaviors. She agrees to an evaluation, which includes observation of her interactions with Michael and his sister. The consultant observes that Joyce reacts differently to Michael compared to Susannah. Joyce seems distressed by his activity level, flinching frequently when he comes near her. She frequently tells him to stop behaviors, but he ignores her. The consultant talks more with Joyce and finds that she is struggling with the idea that her son is like his father, an "abusive man." She has stopped trying to impose any consequences for problem behaviors because sometimes he hits in response. In the classroom, observation shows that he is engaging in frequent problem behaviors, especially when the teacher is working with another child.

A child psychiatrist familiar with early childhood mental health also contributes to the evaluation. Although attention deficit hyperactivity disorder symptoms are noted, given the concurrent parenting issues identified, she suggests dyadic counseling with a parent management training component for Joyce and Michael at a local clinic. At the school, the consultant works with his teacher to identify strategies to help him in the classroom, coordinating with strategies Joyce finds helpful at home. The psychiatrist is also concerned about Michael's language development and recommends department of education evaluation. As a result, he starts to receive speech and occupational therapy services.

Joyce and Michael start meeting with a therapist trained in infant mental health and attachment theory. They explore the moments in sessions when Joyce becomes uncomfortable with Michael. As she understands her own reactions better, she is able to be more consistent with him and recognize him as an individual, not a copy of his father. She notices he seems happier. His teachers report that he is functioning much better in the classroom as well.

## Clinical Pearl

Pre-kindergarten students are expelled at a rate three times higher than other students (grades kindergarten through 12) in the United States (Gilliam, 2005). The behavior problems leading to expulsion sometimes link to issues at home— for instance, children with disorganized attachments, sometimes rooted in distorted views parents have because of their own past trauma, may have more behavioral and emotional difficulties (Lecompte & Moss, 2014; Madigan, Brumariu, Vallani, Atkinson, & Lyons-Ruth, 2016). Relationships provide the scaffolding young children need to learn language, develop problem-solving skills, and internalize social norms, so relational issues also impact on school readiness in nonbehavioral ways.

Preschool consultation models are essentially another version of collaborative care, with placement of a mental health professional in the educational setting. Effectiveness of school-based treatment models has been demonstrated through a number of studies and is discussed in elsewhere in this volume.

Other developmental problems also deserve attention. Often, language/developmental delays and sensory integration problems contribute to behavioral problems. Once the appropriate services are instituted, behavioral improvements soon follow.

Psychiatrists are not always experienced in working with new mothers and infants/toddlers, but those who are committed to public/population health will find that developing a role in the perinatal/early childhood field offers the exciting possibility of true preventive mental health care. Child psychiatrists, in particular, can bring expertise to sorting out complex cases when overlapping symptoms make diagnosis challenging.

Although Joyce, Susannah, and Michael still face numerous challenges, Joyce has forged her identity as a strong maternal figure who supports her children and asks for help when needed. She decides to move out of her mother's apartment because she believes this will be emotionally healthier for her and her children. To do so, they needed to enroll in the family shelter system while applying for subsidized housing. The therapist and the school consultant jointly wrote a letter advocating for placement near the children's preschool so their routines would not be unduly disrupted.

## Clinical Pearl

The advantages of collaboration between medical, educational, mental health, and other providers are clear, although implementing this may require transcending funding, regulatory, and information-sharing barriers. Other involved institutions might include child protective services, family shelters, and public assistance entities. Despite the best of intentions, these institutions may fail to mitigate the intensity of stress weighing on families. Clinicians' advocacy is essential, rallying the system around the needs of children and parents whenever possible.

## DISCUSSION

Unfortunately, there are far too many young children whose home and educational environments do not adequately support their social and emotional development. As demonstrated by the case in this chapter, however, there are many possible opportunities for identifying those families who need support. Women's health and pediatric providers are uniquely positioned for early identification of problems because they interact with mothers and other caregivers during prenatal care and with parents and young children during frequent well-baby visits. Maternal depression screening is well supported by evidence, and review of parental history for adverse childhood experiences is a promising practice for identifying those dyads most at risk for social–emotional problems, providing an opportunity for intervention before problems actually develop (Briggs et al., 2014). Screening for early childhood social–emotional development in pediatric practices is another way to identify problems early, and it dovetails well with developmental monitoring that is already standard of care. A plan for dealing with positive screens is also essential to effective implementation.

A number of established tools are available for social–emotional screening. Some were detailed previously for maternal depression screening; Table 8.2 lists some of the commonly used instruments for young children. In addition, the table lists examples of evidence-based treatments for therapeutic work with parents and young children. Because of the contextual nature of most early childhood mental

*Table 8.2* EXAMPLES OF SCREENING INSTRUMENTS AND TREATMENTS FOR YOUNG CHILDREN

| Screening Instrument | Age Range | For More Information |
|---|---|---|
| Baby Pediatric Symptom Checklist (BPSC) (Sheldrick et al., 2013) *or* Preschool Pediatric Symptom Checklist (PPSC) (Sheldrick et al., 2012) | 1–65 months | https://www.floatinghospital.org/ The-Survey-of-Wellbeing-of-Young-Children/Parts-of-the-SWYC.aspx |
| Ages and Stages Questionnaire: Social Emotional (ASQ:SE) | 1–72 months | http://agesandstages.com/products-services/asqse-2 |
| Early Childhood Screening Assessment (ECSA) | 1½–5 years | http://www.infantinstitute.org/ measures-manuals |
| **Evidence-based treatment** | | |
| Child Parent Psychotherapy | 0–5 years | http://childtrauma.ucsf.edu/ resources-0 |
| Parent Child Interaction Therapy (PCIT) | 2–7 years | http://www.pcit.org |
| Triple P | 0–16 years | http://www.triplep.net/glo-en/home |
| The Incredible Years | 4–8 years | http://www.incredibleyears.com |
| Attachment and Bio-behavioral Catch-up (ABC) | 0–2 years | http://www.infantcaregiverproject.com/about_us |

health problems, individual play therapy for toddlers or preschoolers is rarely indicated and often not helpful.

The California Evidence-Based Clearinghouse for Child Welfare (http://www.cebc4cw.org) provides brief summaries of various mental health treatments for young children as well as older children.

Early education settings provide another important opportunity for identification and engagement in mental health care. Mental health consultants with appropriate training, such as that offered through the Georgetown Model of Early Childhood Mental Health Consultation (https://gucchd.georgetown.edu), help teachers support the growth of specific children who are struggling while also enhancing classroom social–emotional learning and parent engagement. Preschool programs may also use the standardized screening questionnaires mentioned previously to identify children who are in need of more support so that appropriate referrals can be made.

Public adult and child psychiatrists can play important roles in helping develop the systems for screening and intervention that have been described. They are also well positioned to address the need for coordination among multiple service systems because their training and practice span the medical and psychosocial domains. When the strain on families can be minimized by good coordination and planning, parents can use their energy for what matters most—supporting their young children.

## REFERENCES

American Congress of Obstetricians and Gynecologists. (2015, May). *Committee opinion: Screening for perinatal depression*. Retrieved from https://www.acog.org/Resources-And-Publications/Committee-Opinions/Committee-on-Obstetric-Practice/Screening-for-Perinatal-Depression

Briggs, R., Silver, E., Krug, L., Mason, Z., Schrag, R., Chinitz, S., & Racine, A. D. (2014). Healthy steps as a moderator: The impact of maternal trauma on child social-emotional development. *Clinical Practice in Pediatric Psychology, 2*(2), 166–175.

Cox, J. L., Holden, J. M., & Sagovsky, R. (1987). Detection of postnatal depression: Development of the 10-item Edinburgh Postnatal Depression Scale. *British Journal of Psychiatry, 150*(6), 782–786.

Gilliam, W. S. (2005). *Prekindergarteners left behind: Expulsion rates in state prekindergarten programs* (Foundation for Child Development Policy Brief Series Number 3). Retrieved from http://ziglercenter.yale.edu/publications/National%20Prek%20Study_expulsion%20brief_34775_284_5379.pdf

Kroenke, K., Spitzer, R. L., & Williams, J. B. W. (2001). The PHQ-9: Validity of a brief depression severity measure. *Journal of General Internal Medicine, 16*(9), 606–613.

Lecompte, V., & Moss, E. (2014). Disorganized and controlling patterns of attachment, role reversal, and caregiving helplessness: Links to adolescents' externalizing problems. *American Journal of Orthopsychiatry, 84*(5), 581–589.

Lefkovics, E., Baji, I., & Rigo, J. (2014). Impact of maternal depression on pregnancies and on early attachment. *Infant Mental Health Journal, 35*(4), 354–365.

Madigan, S., Brumariu, L., Vallani, V., Atkinson, L., & Lyons-Ruth, K. (2016). Representational and questionnaire measures of attachment: A meta-analysis of relations to child internalizing and externalizing problems. *Psychological Bulletin*, *142*(4), 367–399.

MCPAP for Moms: Massachusetts Child Psychiatry Access Project. (n.d.). Retrieved from https://www.mcpapformoms.org/About/About.aspx

Olds, D. L., Kitzman, H. J., Cole, R. E., Hanks, C. A., Arcoleo, K. J., Anson, E. A., . . . Stevenson, A. J. (2010). Enduring effects of prenatal and infancy home visiting by nurses on maternal life course and government spending: Follow-up of a randomized trial among children at age 12 years. *Archives of Pediatric and Adolescent Medicine*, *164*(5), 419–424.

Olin, S., Kerker, B., Stein, R., Weiss, D., Whitmyre, E., Hoagwood, K., & Horwitz, S. (2015). Can postpartum depression be managed in pediatric primary care? *Journal of Women's Health*, *25*(4), 381–390.

Sheldrick, R. C., Henson, B. S., Merchant, S., Neger, E. N., Murphy, J. M., & Perrin, E. C. (2012). The Preschool Pediatric Symptom Checklist (PPSC): Development and initial validation of a new social/emotional screening instrument. *Academic Pediatrics*, *12*(5), 456–467.

Sheldrick, R. C., Henson, B. S., Neger, E. N., Merchant, S., Murphy, J. M., & Perrin, E. C. (2013). The Baby Pediatric Symptom Checklist: Development and initial validation of a new social/emotional screening instrument for very young children. *Academic Pediatrics*, *13*(1), 72–80.

Women's and Children's Health Policy Center, Department of Population and Family Health Sciences, Johns Hopkins Bloomberg School of Public Health. (2003). Healthy Steps: The first three years—National evaluation final report. Retrieved from http://www.jhsph.edu/research/centers-and-institutes/womens-and-childrens-health-policy-center/projects/Healthy_Steps/frnatleval.html

# 9

# School-Based Mental Health

MIA EVERETT ■

## CASE HISTORY

Cady is an 8-year-old girl enrolled in a third-grade mainstream education classroom. Her school is located in an urban, working-class neighborhood. She has been referred for a psychiatric evaluation in the school-based mental health program in the context of disruptive behavior and declining academic performance. Cady's teacher, guidance counselor, and principal recommended the referral to the student's mother. The referral form highlights a pattern of aggression toward peers, refusal to complete schoolwork, irritability, and restlessness.

### Clinical Pearl

Schools are an opportune setting for addressing barriers to mental health care. Barriers to care for children and adolescents in community outpatient settings include financial and social issues (e.g., insurance coverage, child care, and transportation), stigma, and lack of community or familial engagement by mental health providers. Common reasons for referrals in schools include disruptive behavior, learning or academic difficulties, mood disorders, and impaired social functioning.

After completion of an intake by a licensed clinical social worker, you meet with Cady's mother at school for the psychiatric evaluation. Before you meet Cady's mother, she misses two appointments with you, one due to the illness of Cady's brother and one because her phone was cut off and she did not receive the call regarding the appointment time. Her mother admits that she was reluctant to provide consent for the evaluation, but she agreed given her fears of child protection involvement. Her mother worries about the stigma associated with a mental health diagnosis.

Cady resides with her 24-year-old biological mother, 5-year-old sister, and 3-year-old brother in a domestic violence shelter. Cady's mother reports a history of increasingly disruptive behavior after the onset of domestic violence between her parents several years ago. The guidance counselor at Cady's prior elementary school filed a report for educational neglect with child protective services last year because Cady missed more than 20 days of school. Cady's mother subsequently separated from her father, and the family relocated to the shelter. She notes that Cady is often withdrawn and sullen. She becomes easily frustrated with her younger siblings; she often hits them for taking her toys or interrupting conversations with her mother. Her mother reports that she has difficulty falling asleep at night and complains of nightmares. She shuts down verbally with any mention of her father and startles easily with loud noises.

Cady's mother recalls that Cady exhibited impulsive behavior during kindergarten. Cady has difficulty waiting her turn in lines and has darted into the street while walking with her mother and siblings. Her teachers have noted her difficulty staying seated in class and talking at inappropriate times. Her mother has received daily phone calls regarding Cady's school behavior. Cady has been unable to maintain friendships. She has hit or kicked several of her classmates when provoked. She ignores or talks back to school staff in response to direct commands. She rarely completes assignments, although she demonstrates comprehension of the material. Cady has run out of the classroom on multiple occasions.

Family history is notable for maternal depression. Her mother was sexually abused and placed in foster care as a child. As an adolescent, she was hospitalized several times for cutting and suicidal ideation. Cady's father has a history of substance abuse, several incarcerations for drug possession, and was diagnosed with attention deficit hyperactivity disorder (ADHD) as a child. Cady's mother became pregnant with her at age 16 years. She dropped out of school and moved in with her boyfriend's family. The pregnancy was unremarkable, and Cady was born at full term via vaginal delivery. She met her developmental milestones within normal limits. Cady's mother notes that Cady was difficult to soothe as a baby and was hyperactive. She also had difficulty adjusting to the births of her younger siblings. She attended preschool to second grade at her former school. She transferred to a new school when the family relocated to the domestic violence shelter. Cady has often mentioned that she misses her friends and teachers from her former school. Her mother has limited social support. She receives public assistance and is attending school to earn her GED.

## Clinical Pearl

Classroom observation is an invaluable assessment tool. The frequency and severity of symptoms, triggers and ameliorating factors for specific behaviors, environmental factors, and the nature of peer–teacher relationships are more accurately assessed with classroom observation. Having nuanced information about the educational setting enriches recommendations for treatment, including accommodations and behavioral plans.

Prior to meeting with Cady, you visit her classroom to observe her behavior and social interactions. The teacher reports that Cady is having a fairly uneventful day. She has not engaged in aggressive or dangerous behavior; however, she has refused to participate in classroom activities. The teacher identifies Cady. She is well groomed and thin but adequately nourished. Notably, she frequently kicks her legs, rifles through her desk, or stares out the window during the lesson. She is reprimanded several times by the teacher for failing to pay attention.

At the end of the school day, you meet with Cady in the mental health office. She is initially quiet and guarded; her affect is constricted. You gradually build rapport by inquiring about her interests. She enjoys dancing, listening to music, and playing with dolls. Cady describes her mood as "pretty sad and sometimes grouchy." She does not like going to school because she feels ostracized by her peers. She also believes that her teacher is mean and does not like her. Cady worries about her mother when she is at school. She worries that her father may find out where they live and hurt her mother again. She frequently experiences scary dreams and often feels sleepy during the daytime. She loves her brother and sister but admits that she gets angry when they take her toys. Cady states that her mother often seems sad and spends a lot of time in bed. Cady wants to behave better but has difficulty controlling her anger. She hopes to become a dancer when she grows up. Her wishes are that her mother will not be sad anymore, that her family will have lots of money, and that she will have a best friend.

## Clinical Pearl

Post-traumatic stress disorder (PTSD) symptoms in children may be informed by the relevant developmental stage. Examples of PTSD symptoms in children include re-enacting traumatic events during play, difficulty concentrating, frequent headaches or stomachaches, anger outbursts, regressive behavior, and a fear of dying at a young age.

The following screening measures are completed: the UCLA Child/Adolescent PTSD Reaction Index and the SNAP IV Teacher and Parent Rating Scale. Based on the clinical interview, collateral information, and screening materials, your diagnoses for Cady include PTSD, oppositional defiant disorder, and ADHD.

## Clinical Pearl

The administration of rating scales, in conjunction with the clinical interview and classroom observation, can be a helpful tool in the practice of school-based mental health. Rating scales should be empirically supported with demonstrated reliability and validity. The school-based mental health practitioner may utilize scales to clarify the diagnosis, assess symptom severity and frequency, and track response to treatment. Scales may be designated for the child, parent, or teacher.

You provide psychoeducation regarding the diagnoses to Cady's mother and her teacher. Your recommendations include trauma-focused cognitive–behavioral therapy for Cady, parent management training for Cady's mother, and a psychostimulant trial and an alpha agonist trial pending medical clearance. Additional recommendations include the mother's engagement in mental health treatment, a functional behavioral assessment, a positive reinforcement-based behavioral plan, and completion of a 504 (see Discussion) to provide accommodations in the classroom. The mental health team works collaboratively with school staff and actively engages Cady and her mother in treatment. Specifically, the team educates the teacher about contingency-based behavioral plans and organizational skills. The teacher and treatment team meet regularly to discuss Cady's progress, including her response to behavioral interventions and medications. As the school year progresses, Cady shows gradual improvement in her behavior, academic performance, coping skills, and social interactions.

## DISCUSSION

### Background

The prevalence of diagnosable mental health issues among children and adolescents younger than age 18 years in the United States is approximately 20% (Huffine, 2012). As the scope is broadened, the rates of social, emotional, and behavioral problems among children and adolescents exceed that prevalence. At least 50% of young people in urban schools display significant emotional and behavioral problems (Adelman & Taylor, 2006). Only 20% of children in need of services receive care in the United States, and fewer still receive services from child and adolescent psychiatrists (Huffine, 2012). Educational settings provide the context for 75% of child and adolescent mental health services (Langley, Nadeem, Kataoka, Stein, & Jaycox, 2010). The final report of the President's New Freedom Commission on Mental Health, published in 2003, highlighted the significant public health impact of untreated child and adolescent mental illness; notable goals and recommendations in the report included improving and expanding school mental health programs (Stephan, Weist, Kataoka, Adelsheim, & Mills, 2007). School-based mental health services have shown positive outcomes, including "reduced emotional and behavioral problems, decreased disciplinary referrals, increased prosocial behavior, increased family engagement, improved school climate, and fewer special education referrals" (Stephan et al., 2007, p. 1331).

The provision of school-based mental health services does not just consist of psychotherapy and medication management. School-based interventions may be preventative, either universally offered or individually provided to at-risk students. Programs may promote healthy development and resiliency; support the mental health of families and staff; train school staff to support emotional and academic well-being; and address systemic issues that affect mental health, such as bullying and alienation (Adelman & Taylor, 2004).

The viability of school-based mental health programs is contingent upon securing adequate funding, generally from multiple sources. The primary sources of funding for mental health services are public/government entities, insurance companies, managed care organizations, and private foundations. Both community-based and school-based mental health programs face the challenge of providing services to students without insurance benefits. Grants, rather than fee-for-service reimbursements, are usually required to support mental health promotion or prevention activities, as well as services that insurers generally do not cover, such as classroom observations or teacher consultations (Cammack, Brandt, Slade, Lever, & Stephan, 2014). In the United States, additional federal funding mechanisms for school-based mental health programs include the Individuals with Disabilities Education Act, the Office of Juvenile Justice and Delinquency, and the Department of Education (Cammack et al., 2014).

In addition to psychiatrists, social workers, psychologists, nurses, and counselors may provide services. Parent advocates—parents who have lived experience of raising a child with special needs—can be particularly helpful in this setting. There may be an opportunity to integrate care with a school-based primary care clinic as well. School-based mental health care also involves collaborating with administrators, teachers, and support staff, including paraprofessionals.

Common issues encountered in community school-based mental health include learning disorders, bullying, substance abuse, trauma, sexual and gender identity issues, suicidality, disruptive behavior, and eating disorders. Emotional and behavioral issues may peak at times of transition for students, including the beginning and end of the school year, the transition to new grades/educational levels (i.e., promotion to junior high school from grade school), and changing schools (Adelman & Taylor). Many students in community settings must also contend with additional stressors, including poverty; social isolation; and involvement with social service agencies, including child protective services, residential facilities, and foster care agencies.

## The Psychiatrist's Role

The community child and adolescent psychiatrist may occupy diverse roles in the provision of school-based mental health services. The psychiatrist may serve as a consultant to school staff in addition to providing assessments and treatment for individual students. Psychiatrists provide systems consultation to schools regarding general mental health issues, including creating healthy school environments, valuing diversity, developing prevention programs, and crisis management (American Academy of Child and Adolescent Psychiatry [AACAP], 2005). The successful child and adolescent psychiatrist facilitates collaborative and interdisciplinary care with school staff, social service agencies, parent association groups, and community organizations. Moreover, the psychiatrist should become familiar with the roles of school staff, including administrators, teachers, support services, guidance counselors, nurses, social workers, and resource officers.

Child and adolescent psychiatrists are often consulted to provide recommendations for accommodations and special education services. Familiarity with educational legislation is imperative. Educational rights for children with special needs or disabilities are protected under the Individuals with Disabilities Education Act (IDEA), a federal grant statute that provides funding for special education programs for children with disabilities, and Section 504 of the Americans with Disabilities Act, which "mandates inclusion without discrimination for any person who has a physical or mental impairment that substantially limits a major life activity" in programs that receive funding from the US Department of Education. Psychiatric disorders included in the list of IDEA disability designations include autism spectrum disorders; mood, anxiety, and psychotic disorders; learning disabilities; communication disorders; and ADHD/behavior disorders. Students with disabilities protected under IDEA are eligible to receive services outlined in an Individualized Education Program (IEP). The school-based IEP team develops the written IEP in collaboration with the student's parents or guardians. The IEP team must include the parent, special education teacher, general education teacher if applicable, evaluator, and a school district representative. Optional participants include the child and specialists, such as a parent advocate or disability expert. The IEP is reviewed annually; parents may request a review of the IEP or request changes at any time.

## Treatment and Interventions

The school-based child and adolescent psychiatrist should provide evidence-based treatment recommendations informed by biological, social, and psychological factors after completing a thorough psychiatric evaluation. The recommendations may include, but are not limited to, psychopharmacology, medical or neurological evaluations, individual, family or group psychotherapy, referrals to social service agencies, classroom accommodations, individualized education program evaluations, parenting and educator support, and psychoeducational or neuropsychological testing.

The consulting school-based psychiatrist may recommend completion of a Functional Behavioral Assessment (FBA) and Behavioral Intervention Plan (BIP) for children who exhibit disruptive behavior. The FBA and BIP may be requested as a component of an IEP or as an accommodation under Section 504. Members of the school's IEP team complete the FBA and BIP. The IEP team generally includes a school psychologist. The FBA highlights the precipitating, contextual, and perpetuating factors of disruptive behavior; the BIP specifies behavioral goals and interventions to support the student's achievement of behavioral goals (AACAP, 2005). Evidence-based interventions for disruptive behavior, such as parent management training, may be delivered effectively in the school setting. The Collaborative Life Skills program is an example of a school-implemented psychosocial intervention for children with ADHD (Pfiffner et al., 2016).

The recommendations should address fostering a safe school environment for students and staff, which may include a welcoming atmosphere, a healthy physical environment, collaborative decision-making, a no tolerance policy regarding bullying, social support for students and staff, and "fostering intrinsic motivation for learning and teaching" (Adelman & Taylor, 2004, p. 11). The PAX Good Behavior Game, a simple classroom-based intervention offered by trained teachers, has evidence of a wide range of positive health and social outcomes for children served, and it is gradually being adopted by schools throughout North America (Bradshaw, Zmuda, Kellam, & Ialongo, 2009).

The concepts of resilience and restoration of normal development are considered central to a recovery-oriented approach to public child and adolescent psychiatry (Huffine, 2012). The recovery-oriented approach is person centered and builds on the strengths of the student and the family; community supports and coping skills are optimized and psychosocial/environmental stressors are stabilized with an emphasis on improving health and wellness rather than treating pathology. Features of culturally responsive care include addressing barriers to care, recognizing cultural bias and taking an inquisitive approach to others' culture, conducting evaluations in the family's primary language, evaluating for a history of immigration-related trauma or exposure to community violence, and providing treatment in familiar community settings (Pumariega et al., 2013).

Children and adolescents with behavioral, emotional, and developmental problems are largely underserved. Community child and adolescent psychiatrists practicing in educational settings are uniquely positioned to address the public health issue of childhood mental illness, circumventing barriers to care, including stigma and access issues. The school setting is a natural environment for the child and his or her caregivers that alleviates the burden of travel costs, missed school days or workdays, and finding childcare for compliance with clinic-based treatment. School-based mental health programs facilitate frequent and substantive points of contact between the treatment team and educators. Practitioners have more opportunities to complete classroom observations, which is an invaluable tool for assessing behavioral, academic, and social/emotional functioning.

Fidelity to the principles of public psychiatry is an essential quality of psychiatrists practicing in urban, multicultural, disadvantaged, and often traumatized communities. Transformative care can be wrought with a hopeful, strengths-based approach to mental health care that is culturally humble, systems-oriented, and ultimately empowers youth and their families.

## HELPFUL RESOURCES

Massachusetts General Hospital School Psychiatry Program:
http://www.massgeneral.org/psychiatry/services/treatmentprograms.aspx?id=1944
UCLA School Mental Health Project: http://smhp.psych.ucla.edu
University of Maryland School of Medicine, Center for School Mental Health: https://csmh.umaryland.edu
US Department of Education, Office for Civil Rights, "Protecting Students with Disabilities": http://www2.ed.gov/about/offices/list/ocr/504faq.html

## REFERENCES

Adelman, H., & Taylor, L. *A center brief . . . Integrating mental health in schools: Schools, school-based centers, and community programs working together.* Center for Mental Health in Schools at UCLA. Retrieved from http://smhp.psych.ucla.edu/pdfdocs/briefs/integratingbrief.pdf. Accessed October 18, 2015.

Adelman, H., & Taylor, L. (2004). *Mental health in urban schools.* National Institute for Urban School Improvement. Retrieved from http://smhp.psych.ucla.edu/publications/47%20Mental%20Health%20in%20Urban%20Schools.pdf. Accessed October 10, 2015.

Adelman, H., & Taylor, L. (2006). Special report on child mental health: Mental health in schools and public health. *Public Health Reports, 121,* 294–298.

American Academy of Child and Adolescent Psychiatry. (2005). Practice parameter for psychiatric consultation to schools. *Journal of the American Academy of Child and Adolescent Psychiatry, 44*(10), 1068–1084.

Bradshaw, C. P., Zmuda, J. H., Kellam, S. G., & Ialongo, N. S. (2009). Longitudinal impact of two universal preventive interventions in first grade on educational outcomes in high school. *Journal of Educational Psychology, 101*(4), 926–937.

Cammack, N., Brandt, N., Slade, E., Lever, N., & Stephan, S. (2014). Funding expanded school mental health programs. In M. D. Weist, N. A. Lever, C. P. Bradshaw, & J. S. Owens (Eds.), *Handbook of school mental health: Research, training practice and policy* (pp. 17–30). New York, NY: Springer. doi:10.1007/978-1-4614-7624-5_2

Huffine, C. (2012). Child and adolescent community psychiatry. In H. L. McQuistion, W. E. Sowers, J. M. Ranz, & J. M. Feldman (Eds.), *Handbook of community psychiatry* (pp. 473–483). New York, NY: Springer. doi:10.1007/978-1-4614-3149-7_38

Langley, A., Nadeem, E., Kataoka, S., Stein, B., & Jaycox, L. (2010). Evidence-based mental health programs in schools: Barriers and facilitators of successful implementation. *School Mental Health, 2,* 105–113.

Pfiffner, L., Rooney, M., Haack, L., Villodas, M., Delucchi, K., & McBurnett, K. (2016). A randomized controlled trial of a school-implemented school–home intervention for attention-deficit/hyperactivity disorder symptoms and impairment. *Journal of the American Academy of Child and Adolescent Psychiatry, 55*(9), 762–770.

Pumariega, A., Rothe, E., Mian, A., Carlisle, L., Toppelberg, C., Harris, T., . . . Smith, J. (2013). American Academy of Child and Adolescent Psychiatry Committee on Quality Issues. *Journal of the American Academy of Child and Adolescent Psychiatry, 52*(10), 1101–1114.

Stephan, S., Weist, M., Kataoka, S., Adelsheim, S., & Mills, C. (2007). Transformation of children's mental health services: The role of school mental health. *Psychiatric Services, 58*(10), 1330–1338.

# 10

# Adolescence

RACHEL MANDEL AND RUTH GERSON ■

## CASE HISTORY

Diamond is a 15-year-old girl who was sent to the emergency room (ER) from school after she threatened to kill her teacher. She flipped a desk and punched a wall, but she did not physically attack anyone. She could not be verbally de-escalated, so she was handcuffed by police and transported by ambulance. Her mother was called and met her in the ER. By the time you are consulted, several hours after the incident, she is calm. Diamond tersely insists she is "fine," seems irritated at your questions, and reports the incident as "not that serious." Her mother, however, reports that for the past 6 months, her grades have been falling and she has had increasing behavioral problems, including truancy, breaking curfew, and smoking marijuana. They recently moved into a shelter. When her mother took Diamond to see her pediatrician, he prescribed risperidone and diagnosed mood disorder. Diamond stopped the medication because it made her "sleepy and hungry."

You explain the protocol for the evaluation, treating Diamond and her mother with equal importance and empathy. You allow Diamond to charge her cell phone while you speak with her mother, but you also review the area rules in order to develop rapport and mutual respect.

### Clinical Pearl

When assessing adolescents, little is as it seems at first glance. An adolescent who is brusque and angry on the surface may be sad, anxious, or scared inside. Building rapport and working to understand the adolescent's experience and perspective is key. An accurate diagnosis also requires understanding the child's family context, academic setting and services, community and social environment, and romantic relationships. Access to safe housing, sufficient food, and appropriate treatment is not a given, although adolescents may minimize these difficulties to avoid feelings of shame and vulnerability.

Diamond's mother reports that Diamond was the product of a healthy, full-term pregnancy and delivery. She reached normal developmental milestones and was a happy child. Diamond is the oldest of four children, and she had always been quiet and responsible. She never got into trouble in elementary school, although she was a C student; her teachers said she could do better, but she did not seem very interested in schoolwork. Diamond reached full pubertal development before her classmates in middle school, and she was thus bullied by peers. Her grades declined, and she was held back 1 year, finally able to pass with the help of tutors in a community afterschool program.

### Clinical Pearl

A student who has always been "average" with comments that she "could do better" may have an undiagnosed learning disability or attention deficit hyperactivity disorder (ADHD). Being held back for failing grades is a major red flag. The inattentive subtype of ADHD is often missed, particularly in girls and older children, because teachers expect youth with ADHD to be hyperactive.

Diamond's father was in and out of jail and was murdered when she was 9 years old. Diamond's mother began to struggle with alcohol use, lost her job and then their apartment, and the children were briefly placed in foster care. Although she is working again now, they have struggled financially and remain in a homeless shelter, and Child Protective Services is still involved. Diamond's mother also suspects that the children witnessed and possibly experienced violence while in foster care.

### Clinical Pearl

Sudden loss of a loved one, parental substance abuse, and removal from home and placement in foster care can all be traumatic. Traumatic stress has various manifestations, including post-traumatic stress disorder (PTSD). Depression is the most common consequence of traumatic stress in children and adolescents, and it often presents with irritability rather than depressed mood. Depression and PTSD in youth are underdiagnosed because families may not be aware of the child's internal experience. Youth exposed to traumatic stress may use drugs and alcohol to manage traumatic memories and flashbacks, and they may have temper outbursts when reminders of the trauma trigger anxiety. Adolescents rarely spontaneously discuss their trauma because it is painful and shameful, and traumatized adolescents may have difficulty expressing their emotions. Careful, direct, open-ended questions about trauma exposure are important. Adolescents should be asked about physical and sexual abuse, neglect, bullying, sudden loss of a loved one, parental substance abuse, and community violence.

Diamond's mother states that Diamond started having academic problems in the ninth grade. She could not get extra help after school as she had in middle school. She started skipping school, and she was befriended by other teens who did the same. Her mother thinks they are a bad influence because she has seen pictures of them on social media, scantily clad, smoking and drinking. Diamond complains that her mother is too strict, that the shelter curfew is unfair, and that they have been there too long.

### Clinical Pearl

Adolescents engaging in risky behaviors often misperceive that "everyone is doing it." Youth who binge drink and use marijuana may believe that all adolescents do this regularly, when in fact only 41% of teens have used alcohol and 26% have used marijuana in the past year (Wadley, 2014). Letting adolescents know that these behaviors are not as common as they think is important in enhancing motivation to change.

Per the teacher's report, on the day of the ER visit, the class was taking a math midterm, and many students finished the test quickly and began chatting despite directives to remain quiet. Diamond struggled with the test and grew frustrated by the minor disruptions. One boy mocked her for being "slow," which led to her cursing at him.

### Clinical Pearl

Adolescents with behavioral problems at school are often struggling academically and socially. Adolescents with unmet learning needs often become frustrated by their inability to complete the work, and they may have outbursts or skip school. Teasing by peers worsens the frustration.

The teacher stepped between them to intervene and put his hands on her shoulders to comfort her, but this worsened the situation. The teacher called for security and dismissed the rest of the students as Diamond became verbally threatening and flipped the desk. Once security arrived, she punched the wall and would not accompany them out of the room until police came and handcuffed her.

### Clinical Pearl

Youth who have experienced trauma or abuse are often triggered by unexpected physical contact. Even if a peer bumps into them accidentally, it can trigger trauma flashbacks and lead them to feel threatened and lash out. When approaching an agitated youth, verbal calming strategies should be used. If physical contact is needed for safety, the adult should tell the youth in a calm, clear voice that he or she will be touching the youth—where and why.

You meet with Diamond alone, maintaining professional demeanor but speaking in a casual, conversational manner. She is respectful but guarded, so you ease her into the interview by commenting on her colorful sneakers. You tell her you are interested in her version of events.

Diamond first focuses on the boy who "provoked" her and how "annoying" everyone at school is to her. You empathize, noting that her teacher seems to care about her. She then softens and expresses regret for "getting out of control." She says that this teacher has tried to help her, but she just cannot grasp the material and does not think she can catch up. She wakes up early to travel the extra hour to school from the shelter. In the evenings, she helps with her siblings and chores, so there is little time for schoolwork. There is no quiet space to work, which makes her feel frustrated and irritated. She often goes outside to find friends, who make her feel better. Together, you identify a cycle of feeling overwhelmed by school and family responsibilities resulting in escapism with friends, which leads to falling farther behind. Diamond has insight into this being a poor long-term strategy, but she does not know what else to do. She is able to talk about the negative influence that substances have had on her family, and she is open to finding more adaptive coping strategies. You do a complete psychiatric review of systems, and you determine that Diamond is not an immediate danger to herself or others and does not require inpatient admission. You bring Diamond's mother back in to discuss outpatient options.

You discuss individual and family therapy and referral options. You also recommend after-school programs in their community for educational and recreational supports. You facilitate discussion about schedules, rules, and curfew. You assist Diamond's mother in writing a simple letter to request a psychoeducational evaluation for a possible learning disorder. You provide a list of local legal services to assist with permanent housing and educational advocacy.

Diamond's mother asks about the prior diagnosis of "mood disorder" and medication. You provide an alternative diagnosis of adjustment disorder, given the direct correlation of mood and behavioral disturbance to the extensive psychosocial stressors that Diamond has been experiencing. You encourage the family to follow up with outpatient resources for longitudinal assessment. You discuss the recommendation for psychotherapy alone in treatment of adjustment disorder, although if PTSD and depressive symptoms were to escalate, medication might be helpful.

## DISCUSSION

### Background

Adolescence is a time of peak physical health but also of significant emotional stress. Suicide is the third leading cause of death among 15- to 19-year-olds, and many psychiatric illnesses, including major depression, schizophrenia, and bipolar disorder, can begin in adolescence. Adolescents are particularly vulnerable to psychiatric illness because of biological (i.e., hormonal changes) and psychosocial (i.e., increasing academic demands and social complexity) changes affecting the developing brain. Their increasing independence from family means that parents may not recognize the insidious onset of symptoms. Adolescents with a first episode of psychosis, for example, can go 2 years before they are brought to a physician because parents may attribute changes to typical adolescent moodiness, experimentation with drugs, or the influence of the "wrong crowd" (Marshall et al., 2005). It is difficult to look past adolescent bravado to understand what symptoms are part of "normal" development, what are secondary to environmental stresses, and what are due to primary psychiatric illness. Often, a teen's presentation is a mix of all three.

### Systems Challenges

Adolescents are usually involved in multiple service systems, including at least the school system, but also child welfare, housing, community programs, case management, mental health, or programs for youth with intellectual or developmental disabilities. Although this range of systems should provide a rich menu of supports, it often leads to fragmented care. The clinician who can understand these systems and perceive the big picture can provide leadership in organizing care.

## SCHOOLS

The transition from elementary to middle and then high school mirrors the exciting and chaotic transition into adolescence. Teens are allowed more independence but also more responsibility in terms of schoolwork, exams, peer pressure, and family obligations. Kids who are already at risk can get completely lost in high school without extensive support. Truancy, failures, and suspensions are red flags indicative of underlying problems and not simply adolescent indifference or laziness.

Learning disorders should always be considered in a child who is struggling academically, especially one who has repeated a grade. In the United States, the Individuals with Disabilities Education Improvement Act entitles every child to a free appropriate public education in the least restrictive environment until age 21 years or achievement of a high school diploma. Every school is required to perform psychoeducational testing when a parent requests it. If disabilities are found on testing, then an Individualized Educational Plan (IEP) designates the services that will be provided for the child. The IEP should be reviewed annually and evaluations repeated triennially. Although the IEP is mandated regardless of where the family moves in the United States, sometimes reviews are delayed or missed during school transitions.

Although the special education system is supposed to be user-friendly for parents, with online and printed resources as well as a local "parent member" available in every district to assist, it can still be quite confusing. Anyone working with children needs to understand the system in order to advocate for families and should review the child's evaluations, IEPs, and report cards with parents.

## CHILD WELFARE

A majority of youth in the child welfare system have been exposed to some degree of trauma, and placement in itself can be traumatic. Many have significant mental health concerns due to this exposure, but few receive treatment. Fragmentation of care is common due to placement transitions, lack of collateral information, and lack of treatment consent. The Adverse Childhood Experiences study showed that childhood trauma predicted chronic illnesses in adulthood (Centers for Disease Control and Prevention, 2014). Providing effective trauma screening and care to youth in the child welfare system may help prevent these chronic illnesses. Evidence-based treatments such as trauma-focused cognitive–behavioral therapy may be indicated (Cohen et al., 2010).

## Making the Correct Diagnosis

The psychiatric assessment of an adolescent is complex. Many major mental illnesses have their start in adolescence, but stressors in the home, school, or social environment can trigger psychiatric symptoms, even in the absence of major mental illness. Understanding the broader context of a teen's presentation is crucial in determining appropriate interventions. An isolated change in behavior may be due to a stressor such as a romantic breakup, conflict with parents, or struggles with college applications. To identify potential triggers, approach the teen with genuine curiosity. For a youth who has self-injured, for example, learn about the events and emotions leading up to the decision to cut, whether it was impulsive or planned, and what function it served. In contrast, a teen presenting with several months of academic decline or social withdrawal, or with repeated self-injury, truancy, or substance abuse, may be struggling with a major psychiatric illness. Clinicians should keep in mind that internalizing disorders (depression, anxiety, and PTSD) are often missed in adolescents because they are not as immediately evident as externalizing disorders.

Adolescence is a period of great cognitive and emotional maturation, but youth accomplish this growth at different rates. An individual may be very mature in some areas (e.g., knowledge and vocabulary) but immature in others (e.g., impulse control or delaying gratification). Adolescents' physical maturity may mask profound immaturity in executive function and problem-solving skills. Youth with intellectual or learning disabilities or ADHD are more likely to lag behind their peers in social and emotional maturity. Psychiatric disorders manifest differently depending on the child's cognitive and emotional "age," and the significance of symptoms or behaviors also differs depending on the developmental context.

## Helping Adolescents Access Good Care

Treating adolescents can pose unique challenges because they are often independent enough to participate in their own care but may not have the right or capability to make decisions completely on their own. Providers must walk a fine line between respecting the adolescent's dignity and maintaining confidentiality, while keeping parents involved in treatment. The teen may be seen alone and then with the parent(s), and the parent(s) may want to meet privately as well. The provider can model and facilitate communication and problem-solving between the child and parent(s) and normalize disagreements. Communication with teachers, medical providers, caseworkers, and siblings can inform treatment and also show the teen that the clinician cares about the teen's life as a whole.

Focusing on a child's and family's strengths supports self-efficacy. Children usually come to adult attention when something negative happens, such as a fight or a poor grade. Families are often under stress and may scapegoat a truculent teen, and teens can reflexively view parents as unfair. Identifying strengths that can help the child and family achieve their goals can assist in developing a course of action, including agreement on appropriate rules and consequences. Setting limits on inappropriate or dangerous behaviors is key to maintaining safety. Basic responsibilities such as attending school and not engaging in illegal activity are non-negotiable.

Adolescents are often involved in a myriad of service systems—at the very least, the school system, and often also mental health clinics, child welfare, shelters, community programs, case management, or programs for youth with intellectual or developmental disabilities. This can lead to fragmented care, and the clinician is often the best person to see the big picture and organize the different services and individuals involved. The clinician may also need to determine when a youth requires more intensive mental health services, such as inpatient hospitalization, day treatment, or residential treatment. Currently, provision of evidence-based treatments such as multisystemic therapy and dialectical behavior therapy is inconsistent across these service programs, but public psychiatrists have taken initiative to implement best practices in a number of systems.

This case illustrates both the challenges of treating adolescents and the potential for substantial impact from even a brief intervention. Many providers shy away from treating adolescents, turned off by their bravado and petulance or afraid of their risk-taking behaviors. By joining with adolescents, providers can break through this querulous shell to help identify their needs and to help parents, teachers, and other providers understand how to assist them toward recovery.

## REFERENCES

Centers for Disease Control and Prevention. (2014). *Violence prevention*. Retrieved from https://www.cdc.gov/violenceprevention/acestudy

Cohen, J. A., and the Workgroup on Quality Issues. (2010). Practice parameters for the assessment and treatment of children and adolescents with post-traumatic stress disorder. *Journal of the American Academy of Child and Adolescent Psychiatry*, 49(4), 414–430.

Marshall, M., Lewis, S., Lockwood, A., Drake, R., Jones, P., & Croudace, T. (2005). Association between duration of untreated psychosis and outcome in cohorts of first-episode patients: A systematic review. *Archives of General Psychiatry*, 62(9), 975–983.

Wadley, J. (2014, December 16). Use of alcohol, cigarettes, and a number of illicit drugs declines among U.S. teens. Press release from Monitoring the Future Study. *Michigan News*.

# 11

# Transition-Age Youth

**JEANIE TSE, LARISSA LAI, AND SHARON SORRENTINO** ■

## CASE HISTORY

Ebony was 17 years old when she moved from a state psychiatric facility to a community residence for young adults. She had been in psychiatric treatment since age 7 years, when she was first hospitalized for aggressive behavior. Since then, she has had multiple hospitalizations and medication trials for bipolar disorder. Ebony had been removed from her mother in infancy due to neglect, and she had not met her father, who had been in prison most of her life. She was physically abused in one foster home and has been in group homes and residential treatment since age 12 years. She denies most of the classic symptoms of post-traumatic stress disorder (PTSD), but trauma has affected her ability to form trusting relationships.

When she first arrived at the residence, Ebony presented as disorganized and impulsive—she slept at odd hours, missing meal and medication times, her room was a mess, and she spent her personal needs allowance on tattoos and electronics. She had frequent loud arguments with peers and staff, sometimes banging on walls and doors and making threats. Staff worried about her—like many of her peers transitioning from state facilities, this was her first time living independently.

In keeping with residence procedures, Ebony began her tenure there by developing a service plan with a case manager, discussing her personal goals, her barriers to goal achievement, and her strengths. Ebony wanted to complete school, get a job, and become part of a permanent family, including exploring the possibility of being adopted as an adult. An ultimate goal would be to transition out of the residence to a more independent setting. The residential staff took time getting to know Ebony and reinforcing that she was welcome. They patiently and consistently engaged and redirected her to focus on what she needed to do in order to achieve the goals she set for herself.

### Clinical Pearl

The term *transition-age youth* (TAY) typically describes people aged 17–25 years who are transitioning from child social services, including foster care, to the adult system. Many have severe behavioral health issues, 75% will drop out of school, and 73% will be arrested 3–5 years after leaving school (Levitan, 2005). Many of these youth become homeless. They are making the difficult transition to adulthood with additional burdens of trauma and mental illness and without the family and community supports that peers outside the social service system have.

Many TAY exhibit behaviors consistent with complex trauma and loss, with poor distress tolerance, problem-solving, and impulse control. They often have attachment and trust issues, needing support to develop healthy boundaries and relationships.

At the same time, TAY are an underserved population. Approximately half as many 18- and 19-year-olds are in treatment as 16- and 17-year-olds (Pottick, Bilder, Vander Stoep, Warner, & Alvarez, 2007). This is partly because they seek independence from authority figures at this developmental stage of identity versus role diffusion (Erikson, 1963). More concerning is the fact that our fragmented health care system, with artificial divides between child and adult health care and few cross-links between child and adult diagnostic categories, prevents TAY from accessing treatment.

Breaking through those barriers and engaging TAY in services requires taking time to establish trust, focusing on their personal goals, and providing "scaffolding" as they take risks and learn the natural consequences of their choices.

Ebony tried numerous medications from age 7 to 17 years before finding relief with clozapine. Clozapine helped her manage irritability and aggressive outbursts, and it stabilized her mood, which typically varied from hypomanic to depressed. Challenges to maintaining this treatment included difficulty adhering to blood work and clinic appointments and the medication itself, as well as a period of mild neutropenia that led her psychiatrist to decline to prescribe clozapine for her.

When she arrived at the residence, Ebony voiced her preference for clozapine. Staff advocated unsuccessfully with her psychiatrist, and they finally consulted the agency medical director, who reviewed the record, discussed the situation with the treating psychiatrist, and recommended a retrial of clozapine. This ultimately required a transfer of care to a new clinic.

Ebony connected well with her new psychiatrist and therapist and was enthusiastic about treatment. However, she often forgot appointments or slept in, and she struggled with getting blood work done before an appointment for clozapine renewal. A system had to be developed to help her remember her appointments, including a wall calendar, smartphone notifications, staff reminders, and communication between the clinic and residence when appointments were missed. Continued challenges led the team to suggest she transfer to another clinic nearer the residence or one with more flexible scheduling, but Ebony wanted to stay with her current providers. The treatment team supported this decision but was consistent in helping Ebony understand that she needed to manage her appointments in order to make this successful. It was a great relief, and a marker of her perseverance, when Ebony was able to move from weekly to biweekly and then to monthly blood work requirements for clozapine.

**Clinical Pearl**

Ebony's motivation to participate in treatment may be exceptional, but the amount of support needed from the team to maintain her connection to treatment is typical for TAY. TAY need providers who will align treatment with their personal goals, be flexible with scheduling and missed appointments, and nurture a capacity for attachment that may have been damaged by past trauma. Some calculated risk-taking in the interest of person-centered care may also be needed, as was exemplified by the choice to retry clozapine despite previous neutropenia. A great deal of inter-provider communication is needed to create an adequate, if not seamless, support system for each young person.

Supporting TAY requires a delicate balance between keeping natural consequences at bay (e.g., issuing a prescription despite a missed appointment to prevent recurrent mood symptoms) and allowing learning from natural consequences (e.g., setting limits regarding how many appointments can be missed before treatment may be put on hold). Achieving this balance may require case conferences between providers who may hold different viewpoints.

When Ebony first came to the residence, she had no consistent relationships in her life, let alone trusting ones. Her ability to establish strong relationships with staff members was a testament to her resilience, given her history of trauma and loss. However, she had difficulty avoiding conflict with peers, even when consistently taking clozapine. She isolated herself to "stay out of trouble." A few romantic relationships only made her feel "used" or maligned in the end, reinforcing her mistrust of peers. The staff's consistent supportive stance, even when she was angry or frustrated, helped her learn to regulate her moods. In particular, the presence of a peer specialist at the residence provided a positive experience with someone closer to her age. Gradually, emotional outbursts and conflict decreased, communication and coping skills increased, and Ebony was able to make strides toward her goals.

**Clinical Pearl**

Ebony's experiences highlight the importance of the presence and support of reliable adults in TAY progress and success. A helpful therapeutic stance includes the following:
1. Consistency and repetition—and repetition! TAY need multiple opportunities to learn and practice skills that will help them succeed in the larger community.
2. "Outside the box" thinking: Traditional approaches are not always appropriate for this age group. TAY need providers to support them in finding multiple solutions to a problem.
3. Developing natural supports and full community integration: TAY must develop a network of natural supports that includes reliable adults, supportive peers, mentors, providers, employers, and family. These connections must link TAY firmly to the larger community—a community that is not defined only by their mental health needs.

Vocational/educational and peer specialists at the residence encouraged Ebony to explore different avenues for education and employment. She had left school in grade 10 and had no work experience. Ebony tried completing high school, a GED program, considered college, participated in an internship program, and applied for and worked at several jobs, including a peer position. Many of these explorations lasted only a week or two, but staff supported her in regrouping and choosing a new path each time.

When Ebony first arrived, healthy eating and physical activity had not been a priority for her—her focus had been on staying out of the hospital. However, although clozapine increased her stability, it also increased her weight. Her treatment team began providing wellness education, using motivational enhancement techniques to encourage her to try new health behaviors. For example, her psychiatrist printed out recipes for baked foods that she might like, and she reported on the recipes after she tried them with the help of residential staff. Her focus had moved from day-to-day survival to achieving the best for her future, and her whole health became very relevant to this aim.

Now at age 21 years, Ebony has moved into a supported apartment and is learning to manage roommate issues. She is trying anew to obtain her GED. She is still taking clozapine, having become excessively irritable the two times she tried to taper it off. However, the dose has been minimized, and she has her blood work done on time without staff prompting approximately 50% of the time. She has become more savvy with dating, which also reflects a more secure sense of self. She maintains contact with a few of the staff from the residence, who remain among her champions as she pursues her goals.

## DISCUSSION

### Background

For TAY, moving out of the youth services system poses unique challenges, beyond those experienced by peers who can rely on parental support. The change is often abrupt, with a dearth of support from the health and social services systems, making it difficult for TAY to obtain housing and income, let alone to pursue education and build healthy relationships (Manno, Jacobs, Alson, & Skemer, 2014; Osgood, Foster, & Courtney, 2010). Negative outcomes are more common among TAY, including legal issues, incarceration, homelessness, and experiencing violence in a relationship (Courtney, Piliavin, Grogan-Kaylor, & Nesmith, 2001; Reilly 2003).

The majority of TAY have experienced abuse and neglect that eventually led to their placement in the youth services system, and trauma is also common during their time in foster care (McDaniel, Courtney, Pergamit, & Lowenstein, 2015). Youth in the foster care system often have attachment problems and emotional dysregulation due to family instability and maltreatment (Harden, 2004). Their adult appearances may be misleading if their childhood developmental needs were not met (Aledort et al., 2011). On the other hand, resilience among TAY has been shown to be predicted by female gender, exiting care at an older age, lower perceived life stress, and higher levels of support from family and friends (Daining & DePanfilis, 2007). Participation in services, skills training, and employment leads to better outcomes and greater satisfaction for TAY (Reilly, 2003).

## Proposed Approaches

### INDEPENDENT LIVING PROGRAMS

The Foster Care Independence Act of 1999 doubled federal funding available for states to provide independent living services for youth transitioning out of foster care, and the 2008 Fostering Connections to Success and Increasing Adoptions Act also increased funding to allow states to provide foster care for youths through age 21 years. Some of this funding was channeled to the creation of independent living programs (ILPs), which include housing, vocational and educational services, mentoring, behavioral health services, permanency enhancement, pregnancy prevention, parenting support, financial literacy, and asset-building support (McDaniel et al., 2015). Trauma-focused cognitive–behavioral therapy, an evidence-based psychotherapy model that addresses PTSD symptoms, is used in various ILPs; its focus on trauma narratives can help TAY to develop a sense of mastery over their traumatic memories (Ford, Kerig, & Olafson, 2004).

One ILP model, the Youth Villages Transitional Living Program, features intensive case management with small caseloads and a treatment manual guiding care. This model has been implemented in six states, and it was evaluated in Tennessee, with 1,322 youth randomized to the program condition or a control group that received only a list of community resources. At 1 year, program TAY had better outcomes in terms of earnings, housing stability, economic well-being, and health and safety, although there were no significant differences in education, social support, and criminal involvement (Valentine, Skemer, & Courtney, 2015).

### YOUTH-DRIVEN APPROACHES

Using a person-centered or "youth-driven" approach values TAY's coming of age as adults: The service provider's role is to assist them to set their own goals and make their own informed decisions, providing guidance to develop skills and establish supports for long-term outcomes (Manno et al., 2014). Conventionally, "cultural competence" means understanding the norms of an ethnic group; "cultural humility" involves an open, learning stance in working with people of another ethnicity. Working with TAY may require the same kind of understanding and openness to behaviors, language, customs, beliefs, and perspectives specific to youth culture (Daining & DePanfilis, 2007). Communicating with young adults in a nonjudgmental way that is coherent to youth culture, including making use of the Internet, texting, and social media, can help the clinician engage fully with TAY clients (Aledort et al., 2011).

Involvement with youth services can be associated with stigmatizing labels that may affect sense of self. Paradoxically, youth with mental health problems may also be held to higher standards: Behaviors such as transient truancy or experimentation with substances that might be attributed to a developmental stage for other youths may be regarded as high-risk for TAY (Youth Power, 2015). Involving TAY in treatment planning and allowing them to have space to explore their own individual strengths, abilities, interests, and identity are key in supporting the development of independence (Berzin, Singer, & Hokanson, 2014).

### HOUSING, EDUCATION, AND EMPLOYMENT SUPPORT

Housing, education, and employment outcomes are interlinked: A high school diploma, job skills training, and employment all tie in to influence whether a young adult can maintain satisfactory housing (Choca, Minoff, Angene, & Byrnes, 2004). Housing services include the provision of subsidized housing and supportive programs that assist young adults in obtaining and maintaining housing in the community (McDaniel et al., 2015). Additional support to learn housekeeping, culinary, and financial management skills is usually necessary to help TAY develop and maintain independent living.

High school completion or equivalency programs, college access, and college success programs are among educational services that TAY need. Social support, school stability, and communication with teachers and school administrators are key to academic success. Innovative education strategies—including competency-based learning, focused on mastering particular subject areas instead of completing a classroom time requirement, and blended and extended learning, using technology to permit youth to learn outside of the traditional classroom and class time—may help TAY to overcome traditional barriers to learning (Rath, Rock, & Laferriere, 2012).

A comprehensive approach to supported employment utilizes ongoing assessment of skills and support needs by a multidisciplinary team, including trainers and co-workers, and on-the-job observations and interest inventories (Carter & Lunsford, 2005). Starting to seek employment at a younger age and high future work expectation portend better outcomes (Burke-Miller, Razzano, Grey, Blyler, & Cook, 2012). Conventional employment programs in the behavioral health domain often promote more technical vocations; helping TAY explore and develop longer term career pathways and professional interests may increase their employment potential in the long term (Berzin et al., 2014).

### MENTORSHIP

Many TAY were pushed to become self-reliant in the context of insufficient social support, and they missed the opportunity to explore their identities, roles, and beliefs that is part of the usual transition to adulthood (Arnett, 2004; Greeson, Garcia, Kim, Thompson, & Courtney, 2015). Social support can be provided in various forms, including instrumental, emotional, informational, and affirmational support—all of which are useful for TAY at different moments in their development. Although research on the effectiveness of formal mentorship programs has been inconclusive, reliable adults are crucial to a TAY's success (Collins, Spencer, & Ward, 2010). Mentorship may help youth become more articulate and open with their emotions; establishing mentorship well in advance of the transition age at 18 years supports development of a long-term relationship (Osterling & Hines, 2006). Assisting youth to develop natural social supports with adults and peers eventually helps them to integrate with their communities (Aledort et al., 2011; Collins et al., 2010).

TAY have only recently been recognized as a particularly vulnerable population, underserved by both the youth and adult health and social systems. Public psychiatrists have an opportunity to use an understanding of systems to work toward policies that help TAY to meet basic needs and move toward independence. Skill in using trauma-informed, recovery-oriented, integrated, person-centered, and flexible care helps these young people to transcend the challenges of their past and achieve their goals.

# REFERENCES

Aledort, N., Hsin, Y., Grundberg, S., & Bolas, J.; The New York City Children's Plan Young Adult Housing Workgroup. (2011). *More than a roof over their heads: A toolkit for guiding transition age young adults to long-term housing success.* Retrieved from http://ccsinyc.org/wp-content/uploads/2011/06/YoungAdultHousingToolkit1.pdf

Arnett, J. J. (2004). *Emerging adulthood: The winding road from late teens through the twenties.* Oxford, England: Oxford University Press.

Berzin, S. C., Singer, E., & Hokanson, K. (2014). Emerging versus emancipating: The transition to adulthood for youth in foster care. *Journal of Adolescent Research, 29*(5), 616–638.

Burke-Miller, J., Razzano, L. A., Grey, D. D., Blyler, R. C., & Cook, J. A. (2012). Supported employment outcomes for transition age youth and young adults. *Psychiatric Rehabilitation Journal, 35*(3), 171.

Carter, E. W., & Lunsford, L. B. (2005). Meaningful work: Improving employment outcomes for transition-age youth with emotional and behavioral disorders. *Preventing School Failure: Alternative Education for Children and Youth, 49*(2), 63–69.

Choca, M. J., Minoff, J., Angene, L., & Byrnes, M. (2004). Can't do it alone: Housing collaborations to improve foster youth outcomes. *Child Welfare, 83*(5), 469.

Collins, M. E., Spencer, R., & Ward, R. (2010). Supporting youth in the transition from foster care: Formal and informal connections. *Child Welfare, 89*(1), 125.

Courtney, M. E., Piliavin, I., Grogan-Kaylor, A., & Nesmith, A. (2001). Foster youth transitions to adulthood: A longitudinal view of youth leaving care. *Child Welfare, 80*(6), 685–718.

Daining, C., & DePanfilis, D. (2007). Resilience of youth in transition from out-of-home care to adulthood. *Children and Youth Services Review, 29*(9), 1158–1178.

Erikson, E. (1963). *Childhood and society.* New York, NY: Norton.

Ford, J., Kerig, P., & Olafson, E. (2004). *Evidence-informed interventions for posttraumatic stress problems with youth involved in the juvenile justice system.* National Child Traumatic Stress Network. Retrieved from http://www.nctsn.org/sites/default/files/assets/pdfs/trauma_focused_interventions_youth_jjsys.pdf

Greeson, J. K., Garcia, A. R., Kim, M., Thompson, A. E., & Courtney, M. E. (2015). Development and maintenance of social support among aged out foster youth who received independent living services: Results from the Multi-Site Evaluation of Foster Youth Programs. *Children and Youth Services Review, 53*, 1–9.

Harden, B. J. (2004). Safety and stability for foster children: A developmental perspective. *The Future of Children, 14*, 31–47.

Levitan, M. (2005). *Out of school, out of work . . . out of luck? New York City's disconnected youth.* Retrieved from http://betterfutures.fcny.org/betterfutures/out_of_school_out_of_luck.pdf

Manno, M., Jacobs, E., Alson, J., & Skemer, M. (2014). *Moving into adulthood: Implementation findings from the Youth Villages Transitional Living evaluation.* Retrieved from http://www.mdrc.org/sites/default/files/Youth%20Villages_Full%20Report.pdf

McDaniel, M., Courtney, M. E., Pergamit, M. R., & Lowenstein, C. (2015). *Preparing for a "next generation" evaluation of independent living programs for youth in foster* care: *Project overview* (OPRE Report No. 2014-71). Washington, DC: Office of Planning, Research, and Evaluation, Administration for Children and Families, US Department of Health and Human Services.

Osgood, D. W., Foster, E. M., & Courtney, M. E. (2010). Vulnerable populations and the transition to adulthood. *The Future of Children, 20*(1), 209–229.

Osterling, K. L., & Hines, A. M. (2006). Mentoring adolescent foster youth: Promoting resilience during developmental transitions. *Child & Family Social Work, 11*(3), 242–253.

Pottick, K. J., Bilder, S., Vander Stoep, A., Warner, L. A., & Alvarez, M. F. (2007). US patterns of mental health service utilization for transition-age youth and young adults. *Journal of Behavioral Health Services and Research, 35*(4), 373–389.

Rath, B., Rock, B., & Laferriere, A. (2012). *Helping over-age, under-credited youth succeed: Making the case for innovative education strategies.* Our Piece of the Pie. Retrieved from http://www.taysf.org/wp-content/uploads/2014/08/Hekping-Over-Age-Under-Credited-Youth-Succeed.pdf

Reilly, T. (2003). Transition from care: Status and outcomes of youth who age out of foster care. *Child Welfare, 82*(6), 727–746.

Valentine, E., Skemer, M., & Courtney, M. (2015). *Becoming adults: One-year impact findings from the Youth Villages Transitional Living evaluation.* Retrieved from http://www.mdrc.org/sites/default/files/Becoming_Adults_FR.pdf

Youth Power. (2015). *Youth cultural competency.* Retrieved from https://www.youtube.com/watch?v=13uqgQnOJEM

# 12

# First Episode Psychosis

MARC W. MANSEAU AND JAY CROSBY ∎

## CASE HISTORY

Tyler is a 19-year-old man with no prior psychiatric history who lives at home with his parents and just began his sophomore year at a community college. During the first semester of his freshman year, Tyler began to withdraw socially, staying mostly in his room for weeks at a time and only leaving the house to go to the occasional class. Always a slightly above-average student prior to college, his grades began to worsen and he failed a few classes and thus had to repeat them the following semester. Tyler's parents, professors, and classmates began to notice that his personal hygiene had deteriorated. During the spring semester of his freshman year, his professors began to notice that his writing became increasingly disorganized and difficult to understand and that he would often express odd and paranoid ideas unrelated to the assigned topics, having to do with a conspiracy involving federal agents monitoring him for religious reasons through cameras in his room and wiretaps throughout the school. His classmates noticed at times that he seemed to be listening to something that no one else could hear and that he occasionally muttered things under his breath in public. During the summer, Tyler remained mostly isolated in his room, and his parents noticed that he began to avoid meals and to lose weight. When asked about this, he remarked, "I don't want them to poison me." On one of the first days of his sophomore year, he suddenly stood up in class and yelled, "They're coming for me. Everyone better hit the floor!" Alarmed, the professor called 911 on her mobile phone, and Tyler was brought to the local hospital and admitted to the psychiatric unit on an involuntary basis, where he was started on risperidone.

### Clinical Pearl

A first episode of psychosis (FEP) is defined as the first time when someone experiences positive symptoms (i.e., hallucinations, delusions, and disorganized thinking) that meet *Diagnostic and Statistical Manual of Mental Disorders* (DSM-5) criteria for psychosis. The duration of untreated psychosis (DUP) is defined as the period of time between the onset of the FEP and the initiation of adequate treatment (i.e., with an antipsychotic medication). Longer DUP has been associated with negative outcomes, including more severe positive and negative symptoms, worse treatment engagement, and lower psychosocial functioning (Addington et al., 2015). Therefore, public health and clinical interventions to try to engage people experiencing an FEP in treatment as soon as possible have been increasingly prioritized, with a target DUP of less than 3 months (Figure 12.1).

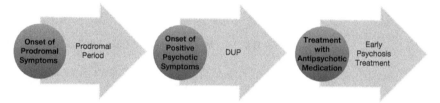

**Figure 12.1** Stages of first-episode psychosis from onset to treatment. DUP, duration of untreated psychosis.

Tyler's risperidone dose was titrated to 2 mg daily and 3 mg at bedtime, and his psychotic symptoms resolved almost completely. After 2 weeks, he was discharged to a new early intervention program for FEP.

Upon admission to the program, a team of clinicians met with Tyler and his family to introduce them to the treatment model and to help Tyler outline his goals. Tyler expressed that he did not have a mental illness but instead believed that "[his] mind was under siege," and he stated that he wanted to take a leave of absence from school. Tyler met individually with the primary clinician, psychiatrist, nurse, and the supported education and employment specialist to begin developing an individualized plan of treatment.

### Clinical Pearl

Based on encouraging findings from investigations of early intervention for psychosis throughout the world, there has been increasing emphasis in the United States on developing specific programs for people who have experienced an FEP. Coordinated specialty care is an evidence-based model that uses a team-based, multidisciplinary approach to flexibly and assertively engage people early in their psychotic illness, with the intention of improving long-term psychosocial functioning and treatment outcomes (Dixon et al., 2015).

Tyler's leave of absence from school left him without daily structure, and he continued to report that he believed he had lost touch with the curious and able part of his mind that had allowed him to succeed in the past. The supported education and employment specialist worked closely with Tyler to help him find a part-time job, which helped him to feel more engaged in the world. His primary clinician met regularly with him in order to understand the impact that his first episode had had on his identity and sense of self-worth.

Although his psychotic symptoms remained under control, Tyler experienced numerous side effects of his medication, including muscle stiffness, akathisia, trouble concentrating, sexual dysfunction, and weight gain. When he considered stopping his medication, the psychiatrist and nurse used shared decision-making (SDM) to help him explore medication alternatives, and they worked with him on exercise and weight loss plans. For example, the nurse reviewed a chart of all possible antipsychotic medications, which included comparisons of likely side effects, and helped Tyler to make a pro and con list for each one. The psychiatrist then reviewed this list with Tyler and guided a medically informed yet personalized discussion of his medication options, including the option of trying no medication. Tyler chose to switch his medication to aripiprazole, which was titrated to 10 mg at bedtime. His weight stabilized and many previous side effects resolved, although he continued to experience akathisia, which responded well to low-dose propranolol.

### Clinical Pearl

People who have experienced an FEP are often more sensitive to antipsychotic medications, in terms of both efficacy and side effects. It is therefore best practice to use the lowest effective dose of a single antipsychotic agent and to employ SDM to include the individual actively in decisions about whether to remain on which medication and at what dose. Side effects of antipsychotic agents at unnecessarily high doses and poor understanding of treatment options are likely major contributors to disengagement from treatment and lower psychosocial functioning over time (Robinson et al., 2015).

Working collaboratively, the team supported Tyler and helped him rebuild his confidence to the point where he could begin to challenge himself with increased responsibilities. Within 6 months, Tyler felt ready to resume his studies, stating, "I feel that my mind is ready to work again." Tyler has not been rehospitalized, and he continues to flourish. He is on track to graduate from community college and wants to pursue a career in human services.

### Clinical Pearl

Even if people who have experienced an FEP struggle to follow all treatment recommendations including medication adherence, they can still be creatively and flexibly engaged in their recovery process. There is evidence that focusing specifically on individuals' life goals, such as work, school, and interpersonal relationships, may be a particularly effective approach (Kane et al., 2016; Lucksted et al., 2015).

## DISCUSSION

### Background

The onset of an FEP can occur precipitously or can be preceded by the insidious onset of prodromal symptoms (e.g., odd beliefs or ideas and social withdrawal) that do not meet criteria for a full-threshold psychotic episode. An FEP can be accompanied by negative symptoms (i.e., avolition, social withdrawal, blunted affect, and anhedonia) and/or affective symptoms (i.e., depressive or manic symptoms), and it may or may not be the beginning of a chronic psychotic illness. An FEP is often, although not always, followed by a first psychiatric hospitalization.

The DUP has become an important concept in research related to early psychosis. Measuring DUP is often complicated. The onset of a psychotic episode is often difficult to ascertain accurately due to deficits in self-reporting and ambiguity in distinguishing prodromal symptoms from the onset of psychotic symptoms. In addition, many people who begin treatment for an FEP rapidly become nonadherent and experience a relapse of symptoms (Kane et al., 2016). Some have argued that time spent untreated early in the course of psychotic illness should be added to the DUP. Finally, the definition of adequate treatment is controversial. For instance, should it be defined as first contact with a mental health professional or first hospitalization for psychosis? Many FEP researchers have settled on time of first antipsychotic administration as the most common endpoint for DUP, although it remains unclear whether this is the best marker of treatment initiation or simply the easiest to measure in a discrete manner.

Measurement challenges aside, it has been fairly robustly established that a longer DUP is correlated with worse clinical outcomes over both short- and long-term follow-up, including more severe positive symptoms, worse response to treatment, a higher risk of symptom relapse, more impairing negative symptoms, and lower psychosocial functioning (Addington et al., 2015; Boonstra et al., 2012; Penttila, Jaaskelainen, Hirvonen, Isohanni, & Miettunen, 2014). A longer DUP has also been associated with deleterious biological markers, such as lower brain-derived neurotrophic factor levels in the central nervous system and loss of cortical gray matter on brain imaging (Rizos et al., 2010). However, other studies have questioned these relationships, especially for functional outcomes, and there does not seem to be any relationship between DUP and cognition— often the most impairing aspect of chronic psychotic disorders (Rund et al., 2016). In addition, it is not entirely clear that the relationships between DUP and clinical outcomes are causal. A longer DUP may be an independent marker of a more severe natural illness course. Nonetheless, the literature linking DUP to clinical outcomes has been strong and consistent enough to make shortening DUP a major clinical and public health priority for those experiencing early psychosis. Internationally, public education and mental health treatment linkage campaigns have been launched to shorten DUP. In the United States, state and local governments have set up specialized treatment programs to better and more rapidly engage people who have experienced an FEP (Dixon et al., 2015; Kane et al., 2016).

## Pharmacology

On average, individuals who are experiencing an FEP tend to have a good early response to antipsychotic medications and to be more sensitive to side effects. Because it is well established that adherence to effective maintenance antipsychotic medication prevents symptom relapse, and that side effects are a major reason for treatment nonadherence, it stands to reason that treatment with the lowest effective dose of a single antipsychotic agent is the best psychopharmacological management approach for FEP. Unfortunately, possibly due to agitation during hospitalization and to pressure to decrease lengths of stay, higher antipsychotic doses and polypharmacy tend to be common upon discharge (Robinson et al., 2015). Therefore, dose reductions and regimen simplifications should be considered once the person who has experienced an FEP is stable as an outpatient.

In addition, although controversial, there is evidence that high-potency typical antipsychotic agents may be more neurotoxic than atypical agents, contributing to problems including more negative symptoms, cortical gray matter loss, increased long-term risk of neurological side effects such as tardive dyskinesia, and lower functioning over time. Due to this risk, atypical agents should be prescribed first, if possible. However, certain atypical agents, such as quetiapine and olanzapine, confer a much greater risk of metabolic problems, such as obesity and diabetes mellitus. These various risks must be balanced carefully, and treatment should be tailored accordingly to the individual's psychiatric and medical needs, but in general, atypical antipsychotic agents with relatively lower metabolic risks (e.g., risperidone, aripiprazole, ziprasidone, and lurasidone) should be considered.

Finally, because medication adherence is both critically important and often incomplete in FEP, initiating a long-acting injectable antipsychotic medication should be considered and discussed early in the course of treatment when appropriate (Subotnik et al., 2015). Due to the complexity and high stakes of adequate treatment with antipsychotic medications in the management of FEP, it is of paramount importance to include the person with early psychosis in the decision-making process regarding whether to take antipsychotic medications and, if so, which agent and at what dose. SDM is an evidence-based way of helping people weigh the risks, benefits, and alternatives and to make informed decisions about their own treatment and recovery, including about psychiatric medications. SDM has been shown to improve treatment engagement and satisfaction, and therefore clinical outcomes, over time (Deegan & Drake, 2006). Although there is risk in allowing someone to choose to forego treatment with antipsychotic medications after an FEP, there is more risk when people disengage from treatment and monitoring entirely.

## Psychosocial Treatment

The emerging standard for FEP treatment in the United States is an evidence-based model called coordinated specialty care (CSC). CSC is a team-based, multidisciplinary approach that encompasses a broad range of interventions that include assertive case management; supported employment and education services; low-dose antipsychotic treatment; family psychoeducation and support; and specialized psychotherapies that address symptom management, social skills, substance use, and suicide prevention. CSC teams are generally composed of four to six clinicians, including a part-time psychiatrist and nurse, and often a peer specialist. Teams are recommended to maintain small caseloads (30–35 clients) so that they can work intensively with clients and families and provide individualized treatment. The goal is to help those experiencing an FEP to manage troubling symptoms and resume progress toward their life goals and interests (Heinssen, Goldstein, & Azrin, 2014). Central to the model is the idea that teams work flexibly and collaboratively with clients within the framework of SDM in order to promote recovery and limit disability (Dixon et al., 2015) (Figure 12.2).

Historically, people experiencing an FEP have been difficult to engage in traditional mental health treatment settings due to social, institutional, and psychological barriers to treatment. Many young adults experiencing an FEP do not identify as having an illness or are averse to the stigma that often accompanies a diagnosis of a psychosis-spectrum disorder. CSC teams must therefore work creatively to engage these individuals and to put their life goals at the front and center of treatment. This might involve conducting assertive outreach to someone in the community, adopting the metaphor or style of language that a person experiencing an FEP might employ to understand his or her symptoms, or promoting an open dialogue with individuals and family members in order to problem-solve and negotiate conflicts that might arise in the context of their lives. Engagement might occur for a certain period of time almost exclusively through the delivery of a single service, such as supported education and employment, with the eventual goal of getting the person more fully engaged with other aspects of treatment (Lucksted, et. al., 2015). Treatment decisions, however, are always made using SDM, allowing the preferences of the individual to be expressed and integrated along with the recommendations of other team members.

CSC is a novel treatment program that incorporates the latest evidence-based psychosocial, pharmacological, and psychological treatments for FEP. In comparison to standard community treatment, CSC has been shown to improve quality of life, reduce the number of hospitalizations, and promote return to work and school for individuals who have experienced an FEP. However, these findings are more robust for individuals with a shorter DUP, thus underscoring the need to increase the availability of specialized FEP services throughout the United States (Kane et al., 2016).

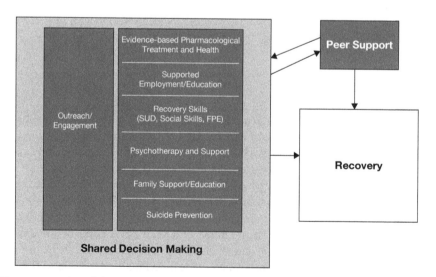

**Figure 12.2** Shared decision-making. FPE, family psychoeducation; SUD, substance use disorders (treatment).
SOURCE: Figure created by Lisa Dixon. Reprinted with permission.

## REFERENCES

Addington, J., Heinssen, R. K., Robinson, D. G., Schooler, N. R., Marcy, P., Brunette, M. F., . . . Kane, J. M. (2015). Duration of untreated psychosis in community treatment settings in the United States. *Psychiatric Services, 66*(7), 753–756.

Boonstra, N., Klaassen, R., Sytema, S., Marshall, M., De Haan, L., Wunderink, L., & Wiersma, D. (2012). Duration of untreated psychosis and negative symptoms— A systematic review and meta-analysis of individual patient data. *Schizophrenia Research, 142*(1–3), 12–19.

Deegan, P. E., & Drake, R. E. (2006). Shared decision making and medication management in the recovery process. *Psychiatric Services, 57*(11), 1636–1639.

Dixon, L. B., Goldman, H. H., Bennett, M. E., Wang, Y., McNamara, K. A., Mendon, S. J., . . . Essock, S. M. (2015). Implementing coordinated specialty care for early psychosis: The RAISE connection program. *Psychiatric Services, 66*(7), 691–698.

Heinssen, R. K., Goldstein, A. B., & Azrin, S. T. (2014). *Evidence-based treatment for first episode psychosis: Components of coordinated specialty care.* Retrieved from http://www.nimh.nih.gov/health/topics/schizophrenia/raise/nimh-white-paper-csc-for-fep_147096.pdf

Kane, J. M., Robinson, D. G., Schooler, N. R., Mueser, K. T., Penn, D. L., Rosenheck, R. A., . . . Heinssen, R. K. (2016). Comprehensive versus usual community care for first-episode psychosis: 2-Year outcomes from the NIMH RAISE early treatment program. *American Journal of Psychiatry, 173*(4), 362–372.

Lucksted, A., Essock, S. M., Stevenson, J., Mendon, S. J., Nossel, I. R., Goldman, H. H., . . . Dixon, L. B. (2015). Client views of engagement in the RAISE connection program for early psychosis recovery. *Psychiatric Services, 66*(7), 699–704.

Penttila, M., Jaaskelainen, E., Hirvonen, N., Isohanni, M., & Miettunen, J. (2014). Duration of untreated psychosis as predictor of long-term outcome in schizophrenia: Systematic review and meta-analysis. *British Journal of Psychiatry, 205*(2), 88–94.

Rizos, E. N., Michalopoulou, P. G., Siafakas, N., Stefanis, N., Douzenis, A., Rontos, I., . . . Lykouras, L. (2010). Association of serum brain-derived neurotrophic factor and duration of untreated psychosis in first-episode patients with schizophrenia. *Neuropsychobiology, 62*(2), 87–90.

Robinson, D. G., Schooler, N. R., John, M., Correll, C. U., Marcy, P., Addington, J., . . . Kane, J. M. (2015). Prescription practices in the treatment of first-episode schizophrenia spectrum disorders: Data from the national RAISE-ETP study. *American Journal of Psychiatry, 172*(3), 237–248.

Rund, B. R., Barder, H. E., Evensen, J., Haahr, U., Hegelstad, W. T., Joa, I., . . . Friis, S. (2016). Neurocognition and duration of psychosis: A 10-year follow-up of first-episode patients. *Schizophrenia Bulletin, 42,* 87–95.

Subotnik, K. L., Casaus, L. R., Ventura, J., Luo, J. S., Hellemann, G. S., Gretchen-Doorly, D., . . . Nuechterlein, K. H. (2015). Long-acting injectable risperidone for relapse prevention and control of breakthrough symptoms after a recent first episode of schizophrenia: A randomized clinical trial. *JAMA Psychiatry, 72*(8), 822–829.

# 13

# Adults with Serious Mental Illness

**SERENA YUAN VOLPP AND PATRICK RUNNELS ∎**

## CASE HISTORY

Joonhee is a 35-year-old woman who is admitted to your hospital. Police were called after she got into a physical altercation with another woman at a fast-food restaurant. When police arrived, she told them that she was angry because the other woman had been sent by Homeland Security to poison her hamburger. On the inpatient unit, she is initially agitated, but she responds well to olanzapine. The team finds out that she had one prior psychiatric admission with diagnoses of schizophrenia and alcohol use disorder. She had not followed up with the outpatient clinic after discharge. Given her lack of insurance, however, you have no other option but to send her back to the same public hospital clinic.

### Clinical Pearl

Individuals with serious mental illnesses (SMI), such as schizophrenia or bipolar disorder, typically struggle to engage in the variety of available services to help meet their psychosocial needs. Access to insurance, particularly Medicaid, for individuals with behavioral health needs is correlated with an increase in the likelihood of receiving treatment (see https://www.ncbi.nlm.nih.gov/pmc/articles/PMC4693853). Just getting and keeping insurance can be a major challenge for people with the disorganization associated with SMI. For example, many individuals with SMI lose their Medicaid because they do not file the annual recertification. Even for those with insurance, mental health service delivery is often fragmented, with poorly coordinated care across inpatient and outpatient realms.

Joonhee does not follow up at the clinic. Within a few months, her mother, with whom she lives, notices that Joonhee has put blackout paper over her windows and tinfoil over the electrical outlets, which she has done in the past when she has started to become paranoid. She tries to get her daughter to go to the clinic, but Joonhee refuses. Her mother calls the social worker at the clinic, who suggests that she call the local mobile crisis team.

## Clinical Pearl

The mobile crisis team (MCT) is a form of crisis intervention service that was developed in the United States in the late 1960s and early 1970s. MCTs are usually multidisciplinary, with social workers, nurses, psychologists, psychiatrists, and, ideally, peer counselors. The teams aim to provide crisis services in people's home environment, helping individuals receive services they might otherwise not be able to access (Gillig, 1995). MCTs receive referrals from family members, clinics, social service agencies, and the police department. In some areas, MCTs have the legal authority to commit an individual to an inpatient setting. Although data are limited, there is evidence that MCTs reduce hospital admissions and thereby provide cost savings (Sabnis & Glick, 2012). Other types of community-based crisis and emergency services include psychiatric emergency services and crisis residential facilities.

When the mobile crisis team visits Joonhee, she tells them that she is not able to leave the house because she is being tracked wherever she goes and that her life is in danger. She is noticeably thin, and she admits to the team that she has only been drinking water and alcohol and not eating food for fear of being poisoned. The mobile crisis team uses its legal authority to bring Joonhee to the hospital emergency room, suggesting that she be admitted due to inability to care for herself. She is admitted to the same unit she had been on months earlier. This time, the unit is able to get a Medicaid-pending status for Joonhee. With that, the unit is able to refer her to the hospital's partial hospitalization program and apply for a case manager.

## Clinical Pearl

Partial hospitalization is an intermediate option that can help reduce the use of inpatient hospitalization while also providing more autonomy for patients. In some areas configured as intensive outpatient programs, partial hospitalizations are voluntary, outpatient programs lasting weeks to months that provide programming for several hours a day, including occupational therapy, recreational therapy, individual therapy, and exercise groups. Psychiatrists see patients once or several times weekly rather than daily. Partial hospitalizations are often employed to prevent full hospitalization or to facilitate a more rapid step-down from full inpatient psychiatric care (Khawaja & Westermeir, 2010). A meta-analysis showed that partial hospitalization is as effective as full hospitalization for the subset of individuals who do not meet criteria for involuntary hospitalization, and it is also more cost-effective, with higher patient and family satisfaction (Horvitz-Lennon et al., 2001). Continuing day treatment programs, which usually involve 5 days-a-week programming on a longer term basis, are another level of service more intensive than a clinic. New York state also offers a model called PROS (Personalized Recovery Oriented Services), which is more individualized and flexible than continuing day treatment and focuses on helping each individual define and attain his or her personal goals.

Case management is a service typically provided by paraprofessionals or social workers that focuses on building relationships with individuals to support them in engaging with mental health, physical health, and psycho-social services, including supported employment, housing, and financial management.

Joonhee's attendance at the partial hospitalization program is poor, and her case manager has a difficult time establishing rapport with her. Her mother reports that she found Joonhee's pills in the garbage along with empty bottles of vodka. After a month of no attendance, the partial hospitalization program closes her case. Five months later, Joonhee is brought to the hospital. During this hospitalization, the inpatient team manages to convince Joonhee to try a long-acting injectable anti-psychotic. She stabilizes and is given two injections 1 week apart just prior to discharge. Based on her number of admissions, she now meets criteria for assertive community treatment.

### Clinical Pearl

Assertive community treatment (ACT) employs a multidisciplinary team to deliver high-intensity, community-based care for individuals with SMI who struggle to engage in outpatient services and are at high risk for repeated psychiatric hospitalizations. The team typically includes a mix of case managers, substance abuse specialists, employment specialists, peer supports, nursing, psychiatry, and, increasingly, primary care. Teams are characterized by high staffing ratios (typically 10–15 individuals per team member); frequent, community-based visits (at least six per month); and 24-hour access. ACT has been extensively researched, demonstrating substantial reduction in psychiatric hospitalizations, improved housing stability, symptom reduction, and improved subjective quality of life (Bond et al., 2001).

Joonhee takes a strong dislike to two of the ACT team members, but she forms a connection with the peer specialist on the team over their shared love for fried chicken. He is in recovery from alcohol himself, and, using a harm reduction framework, he is very gradually able to get her to reduce her alcohol consumption. Although Joonhee does not like the family specialist very much, she does allow this worker into the home, and the worker is able to provide some support to Joonhee's mother. Joonhee does agree to the injectable every month, but she is noted to have residual paranoia. Although there is no one on the team who has been trained in cognitive behavioral therapy for psychosis (CBTp), the team is able to refer Joonhee to a CBTp group at a community clinic near her house. The team also refers Joonhee to a supported employment program, and she obtains a job at a fast-food restaurant. The employment program provides a job coach who helps Joonhee problem-solve when she gets into disagreements with her co-workers. Although she is not completely sober, Joonhee manages to stay out of the hospital for the next year.

## DISCUSSION

The clinician's goal for every adult with SMI should be recovery, moving beyond symptom control to the promotion of the individual's functioning, autonomy, and sense of purpose. Evidence-based recovery support services include illness management; supported employment, education, and housing; assertive community treatment; and peer-operated services.

The concept of health self-management refers to an individual's ability to manage his or her own illness as an active participant in his or her own care. Several programs have been developed for self-management in behavioral health, including Wellness Recovery Action Plans (WRAP), Neuroscience Treatment Team Partners (NTTP), Illness Management and Recovery (IMR), and Wellness Self-Management (WSM) (Salerno & Margolies, 2012). IMR is recognized as an evidence-based practice by the Substance Abuse and Mental Health Services Administration. The individual can meet with peers or clinicians to go through a series of lessons and/or workbooks that promote informed decision-making and development of the patient's personal goals.

One misconception about schizophrenia is that psychotic symptoms prevent individuals from attaining and maintaining gainful employment. The majority of individuals with schizophrenia want to work, but only 15% of individuals typically attain competitive employment without help. Whether embedded in an ACT team or standing on its own, models of supported employment have shown significant results in increasing workforce participation for individuals with schizophrenia (Mueser & Bond, 2012). The most widely studied model of supported employment is individual placement and support (IPS). In this model, individuals are assigned an employment coach who helps them find and apply for competitive jobs, guides them through the interview process, and then works alongside them once they are hired, both to ensure they get extra support in learning the job and to help fill in for work when they have symptom flare-ups. Compared with the base rate of 15%, IPS increases attainment of employment to more than 50%, and long-term studies show that the vast majority of individuals who attain employment through IPS continue to be gainfully employed many years later.

Psychosis, co-occurring addictions, cognitive deficits, poor executive functioning, and lack of social support all contribute to housing instability for individuals with SMI. For several decades, the primary mechanism for obtaining housing was through the continuum of care (or linear) model, whereby individuals had to demonstrate "housing readiness" by engaging successfully in prescribed treatment programs. From there, they were moved into a highly staffed and structured living arrangement. As they demonstrated specific measures of success, they progressed through a system of housing with increasing levels of autonomy and decreasing levels of supervision, with an end goal of attaining independent housing. The success rate for achieving housing independence in this model was not high (Gulcur, Stefanic, Shinn, Tsemberis, & Fischer, 2003). In the early 1990s, the innovative program Pathways to Housing piloted a novel method for helping individuals with schizophrenia obtain and maintain housing by combining two concepts: *supportive housing* and *housing first*. The program started with the supposition that individuals could not successfully engage in treatment without steady, independent housing. Thus, they arranged for individuals to be "housed first" and then wrapped support services around the new living arrangement. The success was astounding: 88% of individuals in the original study maintained housing for greater than 2 years; even more impressive, this model has achieved identical results in several follow-up studies (Tsemberis & Eisenberg, 2000). Supportive housing paired with housing first is now considered the gold standard for helping homeless individuals with SMI achieve housing independence.

Although a minority of patients with SMI achieve recovery without medication maintenance, for most, maintenance treatment with medication is recommended. Adherence to treatment, and particularly to medication, can be a major challenge. Medication adherence for individuals with psychotic disorders is estimated to be 25–50%; for those with bipolar disorder, it is estimated to be 35–57% (Hartung et al., 2017). Active substance use is a risk factor for poor adherence. Poor adherence leads to increased hospitalization rates (Hartung et al., 2017), an undesirable outcome both for patients and for health care system costs. It is important to remove logistical barriers to adherence, such as lack of insurance and difficulty obtaining medication from the pharmacy. If disorganization and cognitive decline are primary causes of nonadherence, simplification of dosing regimens, the use of long-acting injectable antipsychotics, and the use of pillboxes and alarms may help. Medication side effects are significantly associated with nonadherence; prevention, identification, and management of side effects are crucial (Dibonaventura, Gabriel, Dupclay, Gupta, & Kim, 2012). Many patients with SMI are not adherent due to a lack of insight into their symptoms or illnesses. Establishing a therapeutic alliance, using motivational interviewing, being candid about potential risks in addition to benefits, and using a harm reduction framework are helpful techniques to improve adherence. Financial incentives have also been studied and show some promise in improving adherence rates, although this practice raises multiple ethical issues (Noordraven et al., 2017).

When other strategies to improve adherence have failed, assisted outpatient treatment (AOT) is an option. AOT, also called outpatient commitment, involuntary outpatient commitment, and mandatory outpatient treatment, is a court order issued in civil court mandating the individual to a particular treatment plan. In the United States, 46 states and the District of Columbia have AOT (the exceptions are Connecticut, Maryland, Massachusetts, and Tennessee). Most Canadian provinces have a version of AOT called Community Treatment Orders. AOT laws are most commonly applied to individuals who have a history of repeated hospitalizations and/or a serious history of violence or suicide attempts. Less commonly, AOT is used in some states to try to prevent hospitalizations. Implementation of AOT varies from state to state; in most states, no additional funding resources are provided for AOT, with New York state being a notable exception. A retrospective evaluation of New York state AOT from 1999 to 2007 found that during the first 6 months of AOT, hospitalization admissions were reduced by approximately 25%, and likelihood of admission was reduced even further with additional time on court order. Compliance with medication, as defined by greater than 80% medication possession, increased by almost 50% during the first 6 months of AOT, and it increased by nearly 90% during the subsequent 6 months (Swartz et al., 2010). In addition to mandating that patients be accountable for their treatment, AOT also makes service providers accountable to patients. Detractors criticize AOT as a form of coercion that does not support person-centered recovery.

Although busy community psychiatrists by necessity must often focus on medication treatments, CBTp is a psychotherapeutic treatment well established in some countries (e.g., CBTp is a standard treatment recommendation for first-episode psychosis in England's National Health Service) and gaining more attention in the United

States. Randomized controlled trials of CBTp have shown moderate effect sizes for positive and negative symptoms, with sustained benefits over time (Tai & Turkington, 2009). A central premise of CBTp is that people with psychosis can think logically and can be taught to question their delusions and/or hallucinations. Groundwork is laid to normalize psychotic symptoms as being on a continuum of human experience, and care is taken to discuss with the patient what chronic and acute stressors may have contributed to these symptoms. The therapy is collaborative and focuses on managing and reducing the distress of the individual living with psychosis. CBTp is much more challenging with individuals who have disorganized thought processes.

Individuals who have lived experience with mental illness—peer counselors— are paid professionals who, having experienced significant recovery themselves, enter into intentional relationships with consumers (typically suffering from a similar disorder) to help promote their own recovery process. Their work focuses on acceptance, treatment engagement, and strategies for managing symptoms, as well as the isolation, despair, and demoralization that often accompany them (Davidson, Chinman, Sells, & Rowe, 2006). Separately, consumer-run programs can also leverage the concept of shared community to promote successful recovery. The most studied of these models is the *clubhouse*. In this model, members participate directly in the operation and governance of all clubhouse functions, including finance/budgeting, meal preparation, facility maintenance, and membership. Clubhouses also usually include housing, education, and transitional employment programs, and they emphasize the value of the work-ordered day. The clubhouse model has been shown to improve outcomes related to employment and other recovery metrics (Macias, Berreira, Alden, & Boyd, 2001). Fountain House in New York City is the prototype clubhouse. The International Center for Clubhouse Development has created benchmarks for how to establish effective models, leading to the successful development of thousands of clubhouses throughout the world.

The range of services, interventions, and approaches available to help improve the lives of individuals with serious mental illness is expansive and well studied. For most, however, access to even a part of these services is limited. Often, these interventions do not translate easily into traditional billing categories, making them difficult to sustain. Despite the fact that these services often save money over the long term, payers may be unwilling to increase reimbursement for services that are more expensive in the short term or whose benefits do not result in immediate cost savings for payers. Advocacy to improve the quality and access to care remains an important part of the repertoire for everyone working in mental health.

## REFERENCES

Bond, G., Drake, R., Mueser, K., & Latimer, E. (2001). Assertive Community Treatment for People with Severe Mental Illness: Critical Ingredients and Impact on Patients. *Disease Management & Health Outcomes, 9*(3), 141–159.

Davidson, L., Chinman, M., Sells, D., & Rowe, M. (2006). Peer support among adults with serious mental illness: A report from the field. *Schizophrenia Bulletin, 32*(3), 443–450.

Dibonaventura, M., Gabriel, S., Dupclay, L., Gupta, S., & Kim, E. (2012). A patient perspective of the impact of medication side effects on adherence: Results of a cross-sectional nationwide survey of patients with schizophrenia. *BMC Psychiatry, 12,* 20.

Gillig, P. (1995). The spectrum of mobile outreach and its role in the emergency service. *New Directions for Mental Health Services, 67,* 13–20.

Gulcur, L., Stefanic, A., Shinn, M., Tsemberis, S., & Fischer, S. N. (2003). Housing, hospitalization, and cost outcomes for homeless individuals with psychiatric disabilities participating in continuum of care and housing first programmes. *Journal of Community and Applied Social Psychology, 13,* 171–186.

Hartung, D., Low, A., Jindal, K., Mansoor, D, Judge, M., Mendelson, A., . . . Kondo, K. (2017). Interventions to improve pharmacological adherence among adults with psychotic spectrum disorders and bipolar disorders: A systematic review. *Psychosomatics, 58*(2), 101–112.

Horvitz-Lennon, M., Normand, S. T., Gaccione, P., & Frank, R. G. (2001). Partial Versus Full Hospitalization for Adults in Psychiatric Distress: A Systematic Review of the Published Literature (1957–1997). *American Journal of Psychiatry, 158*(5), 676–685.

Khawaja, I. S., & Westermeyer, J. J. (2010). Providing Crisis-oriented and Recovery-based Treatment in Partial Hospitalization Programs. *Psychiatry (Edgmont), 7*(2), 28–31.

Macias, C., Berreira, P., Alden, M., & Boyd, J. (2001). The ICCD benchmarks for clubhouses: A practical approach to quality improvement and psychiatric rehabilitation. *Psychiatric Services, 52*(2), 207–213.

Mueser, K. T., & Bond, G. R. (2012). Supported employment. In H. L. McQuistion, W. E. Sowers, J. M. Ranz, & J. M. Feldman (Eds.), *Handbook of community psychiatry* (pp. 309–318). New York, NY: Springer.

Noordraven, E. L., Wierdsma, A. I., Blanken, P., Bloemendaal, A. F., Staring A. B., & Mulder, C. L. (2017). Financial incentives for improving adherence to maintenance treatment in patients with psychotic disorders (Money for Medication): A multi-centre, open-label, randomised controlled trial. *Lancet Psychiatry, 4*(3), 199–207.

Sabnis, D., & Glick, R. L. (2012). Innovative community-based crisis and emergency services. In H. L. McQuistion, W. E. Sowers, J. M. Ranz, & J. M. Feldman (Eds.), *Handbook of community psychiatry* (pp. 379–387). New York, NY: Springer.

Salerno, A. J., & Margolies, P. J. (2012). Behavioral and physical health self-management. In H. L. McQuistion, W. E. Sowers, J. M. Ranz, & J. M. Feldman (Eds.), *Handbook of community psychiatry* (pp. 319–327). New York, NY: Springer.

Swartz, M. S., Wilder, C. M., Swandon, J. W., Van Dorn, R. A., Robbins, P. C., . . . Monahan, J. (2010). Assessing outcomes for consumers in New York's assisted outpatient treatment program. *Psychiatric Services, 61*(10), 976–981.

Tai, S., & Turkington, D. (2009). The evolution of cognitive behavior therapy for schizophrenia. Current practice and recent developments. *Schizophrenia Bulletin, 35,* 865–873.

Tsemberis, S., & Eisenberg, R. F. (2000). Pathways to housing: Supported housing for street-dwelling homeless individuals with psychiatric disabilities. *Psychiatric Services, 51,* 487–493.

# The Elderly

DENNIS POPEO ■

## CASE HISTORY

Justin is a 75-year-old man who presented to the medical emergency department of your city hospital with complaints of eye and ear pain. When he reported that his pain was caused by "police satellites using stun guns" to electrocute his eyes and that the "FBI has been putting semen" in his ears, he was sent to the psychiatric emergency room to be evaluated.

Upon examination, Justin was pleasantly cooperative, though slightly disheveled. He reported that he has been wandering through the city feeling depressed about his current issues with the police and the FBI. He stopped the interview to report that he was having trouble hearing. After suggesting that the interview be relocated to a quieter spot, Justin was noted to be gingerly making his way across the highly polished floor.

### Clinical Pearl

#### Evaluation of Older Adults Requires Some Special Care

Although older adults are a very heterogeneous population with regard to abilities, many have sensory deficits that make evaluation difficult (Karp, 2011). As people age, hearing impairment becomes more common. Make sure that the patient can hear you by speaking clearly in a normal tone. Try to avoid conversations in areas with background noise because that can be distracting and can drown out what is said. Speaking when behind a glass partition (even with a hole for sound to escape) can make hearing difficult. Visual deficits can also hinder understanding. Adequate lighting and the use of glasses should be encouraged. Any written material should be printed clearly and in a large font.

Finally, the environment of care plays a role in a successful and safe evaluation of the older patient. Glare from overhead lights on highly polished floors can make the floors look wet and slippery. Chairs without arms can be a risk for falls, and chairs or examination tables that are too low or two high can also pose risks for trips or falls (Chun, 2011).

After having settled into a quieter interview room, Justin reported that he was diagnosed with schizophrenia "years ago" and had taken medications "on and off" his entire life. He noted suicide attempts in the late 1970s and in the 1980s. He noted that his current worries about the police, FBI, and other government authorities are so troubling that he has been planning to jump into the river in order to kill himself.

Justin reported that he was divorced "years ago" and that he used to live in Prosperity Park, an adult home that was recently closed. He noted that he was sent to live with his niece out in the country. Unfortunately, his providers were still in the city, and he had difficulty managing appointments with his new commute. His level of service was dropped from a day program to appointments every other week. His niece had difficulty finding appropriate psychiatric care that would accept Medicare. Justin reports that he misses the groups and activities in the day program, and he says that he has not been able to get medications for at least a month. His niece was unable to be reached at the numbers programmed into Justin's phone.

## Clinical Pearl

### Heath Care Accessibility for Older Adults Can Be Problematic

The US Census Bureau defines older adults as those aged 55–64 years and elderly as those aged 65 years old or older. The population of elderly adults is expected to grow from 48 million in 2015 to approximately 80 million in 2035. During the same time period, the number of persons older than age 85 years is projected to nearly double from 6 million to approximately 12 million (US Census Bureau, 2014). Specialists trained in geriatric mental health are already in short supply, and current projections suggest that we will not be able to meet the increased needs of the older mentally ill (Institute of Medicine [IOM], 2012).

Mentally ill older adults tend to have a lower rate of service use compared to younger adults. This is probably related to a lack of age-appropriate and culturally appropriate services for both the prevention and treatment of mental illness. Unfortunately, services for older adults with mental illness are costly. With cuts to Medicaid and threats to Medicare, many programs simply cannot survive, much less fully serve the needs of this growing community (Cohen & Ibrahim, 2012; Palinkas et al, 2007).

Justin's psychosis, suicidality with a lethal plan, and tenuous aftercare arrangements necessitate an admission. Justin is cooperative with medications and allows the hospital staff to contact his prior treatment providers. He is started on an antipsychotic at a low dose due to the likelihood that he has age-related diminished metabolism in the liver. His medical workup reveals untreated hypertension, and he is prescribed an antihypertensive. He also allows the team to contact his niece, but she remains elusive. The social worker and hospital finance officer assigned to the unit find that she is his social security payee. When questioned, Justin reports his niece takes his check for rent and gives him a $20 per month allowance.

## Clinical Pearl

### Unfortunately, Elder Abuse Happens, and It Is Not Just Physical

There are five major categories of elder abuse: physical abuse, psychological (verbal) abuse, sexual abuse, financial exploitation, and neglect. The prevalence of elder abuse has been described as between 7% and 10%, but these percentages likely represent an underestimation of cases. Because the majority of abusers are family members, older adults are less likely to report abuse, and patients with cognitive impairment may not be able to report abuse to their physicians.

The risk factors for elder abuse include female gender, younger age, low income, a diagnosis of dementia, greater functional impairment, poor physical health, social isolation and lack of social support, as well as residing in a shared living environment. Perpetrators of elder abuse are more likely to be adult children or spouses, be male, have a history of past or current substance abuse, have mental or physical health problems, be socially isolated, be unemployed or have financial stress, and be experiencing major stressors. Caregiver stress, in particular, can be overwhelming, and it increases the risk for elder abuse (Johannesen & LoGiudice, 2013; Lachs & Pillemer, 2015).

All health care providers have a mandate to report suspected abuse to adult protective services, which can assist with legal actions and can apply for guardianship, if necessary.

Justin stabilized psychiatrically, and his niece responded to a certified letter from the social worker that threatened to cut off his social security benefits. She agreed to have Justin return to her home, and he was discharged there. He was referred to nearby psychiatric services and to the local adult protective services for suspicions of financial exploitation.

Two weeks later, Justin returned to the emergency department agitated, paranoid, and disheveled. He was again admitted, and again, his niece was unresponsive to outreach. As Justin stabilized psychiatrically, he reported that he lost his medications and did not want to present to the local treatment provider because he likes coming to the city. He noted that he was not interested in returning to his niece's house because she had not been giving him his allowance. During this admission, the unit social worker was able to change Justin's social security payee. The niece called soon after she discovered this, noting that she believed Justin was "too difficult" to return to her home.

Thus, a new discharge plan was needed. Justin reported that he wanted to stay in the city. Housing options were limited given Justin's diagnosis of schizophrenia. Cognitive testing revealed a minor neurocognitive disorder but no skilled nursing needs, ruling out the possibility of a nursing home referral. He noted that he had tried to stay in a homeless shelter, but he found the rules and procedures confusing. He stated, "It's hard to be mentally ill."

### Clinical Pearl

#### Housing Options for the Homeless Mentally Ill Elderly Are Limited and Can Be Inappropriate

Ten to fifteen percent of the homeless population are elderly. Many individuals currently between the ages of 60 and 70 years are living in poverty and are at risk for homelessness. As the "Baby Boomer" cohort ages, the number of housing insecure elders will increase. Also, middle-aged homeless adults are aging into the elderly age group. Homeless elderly adults tend to have more chronic medical illness compared to their housed counterparts and are more likely to suffer from cognitive impairments. They require significantly more specific services compared to younger homeless adults.

Standard homeless shelters most often do not have the capacity to manage the increased medical needs of older adults. Shelters can be dangerous for cognitively impaired elders both due to environments that were not built with elderly clients in mind and due to the risk for abuse by other shelter residents.

A lack of affordable housing and a lack of service-enriched housing perpetuate the problem of elderly homelessness. Unfortunately, laws meant to protect the rights of people with mental illness, and to prevent them from being warehoused in skilled-nursing facilities and "adult homes," have made it more difficult to place the mentally ill who do not have significant cognitive impairment or skilled nursing needs. Often, it is suggested that these elders would be better cared for in the community, but community services available simply do not meet their needs (Gonyea, Mills-Dick, & Bachman, 2010; National Coalition for the Homeless, 2009). All states have a designated agency or bureau on aging that is responsible for addressing these issues and may be able to provide referral services.

Fortunately, the inpatient social worker was able to secure Justin a rare spot in a residential care facility, paid for by his social security income. She also applied for a case manager who will help him navigate his new living situation and set up community-based services such as transportation to his appointments and shopping assistance.

## DISCUSSION

The population of adults aged 65 years or older is expected to reach 74 million individuals by 2030 (US Census Bureau, 2014). Mental illness, including memory problems, is expected to affect more than 15 million of those people (Palinkas et al., 2007). Not only will this massive demographic shift overwhelm the health care system, but also it will stretch already thinning public and community mental health resources for older adults with mental illness (IOM, 2012). There are and will be many areas for intervention and opportunities for public psychiatrists to make a difference.

In order to begin to meet the needs of older adults with mental illness, we must define those needs. Palinkas et al. (2007) attempted to define those needs in San Diego County, California, by identifying and interviewing stakeholders, including health care providers, social service providers, caregivers, and consumers. They found that the most important gap in service was an absence of age-appropriate or culturally appropriate services. This was closely followed by a lack of information on how to access existing services, which included difficulty in the financing of and transportation to those services. Finally, coordination of those services with physical health and social services was found to be lacking.

Creating an age-appropriate service for older adults must take into account limitations in time and mobility. Individuals in this age group who have mental health issues often also have physical health issues and social service needs, resulting in frequent service appointments (Horgan et al., 2009). Integrating mental health services into primary care clinics or social service organizations can resolve some of these issues (Bartels, 2003). There is evidence that this type of program can be cost-saving, but many of these types of collaborative programs are not yet reimbursed by traditional insurance (Cohen & Ibrahim, 2012).

Age-appropriate care must balance the autonomy of the individual with the needs of caregivers and other stakeholders involved in their health care (Horgan et al., 2009). For instance, structuring interactions to last longer than the typical amount of time set aside for a visit of a younger adult is often needed, but this can be difficult to accomplish in a busy medical practice (Karp, 2011). The environment of care needs to be carefully structured and designed to meet the needs of older adults (Chun, 2011). Caregivers may need to be involved in visits, care coordination, and decision-making, although their involvement may place additional strain on their time and caregiving capacity (Wolff, Spillman, Freedman, & Kasper, 2016). Communication between multiple providers, patients, and caregivers needs to flow easily, although a patient may not want information to be shared in all instances. Caregiver support and recognition of caregiver burden must be an integral part of any intervention for elder mental health (Adelman, Tmanova, Delgado, Dion, & Lachs, 2014).

Cognitive impairment is often a major factor when planning services for the elderly. The prevalence of cognitive impairment in individuals aged 65 years is approximately 1%, and that prevalence doubles every 5 years (Brookmeyer, Johnson, Ziegler-Graham, & Arrighi, 2007). When considering individuals with cognitive impairment and symptoms of mental illness, the "chicken or the egg" conundrum occurs: Many mental illnesses (e.g., schizophrenia and bipolar disorder) result in cognitive dysfunction (Green, 2006), and individuals who are cognitively impaired commonly have behavioral and psychiatric symptoms. Mackin and Areán (2009) tested 52 older adults previously diagnosed with severe mental illness who were participating in community mental health treatment and found that 60% suffered cognitive impairment.

Cognitive screening is recommended for all adults older than age 70 years at least once a year. Numerous screening instruments have been validated (Morley et al., 2015), but not specifically in populations with mental illness. For instance, the Mini-Mental State Examination has been shown to underestimate cognitive impairment in psychiatric patients (Faustman, Moses, & Csernansky, 1990). Cognitively impaired elders have more difficulty adhering to treatment plans (including relatively "simple" plans such as taking medications), navigating to appointments, and maintaining independence (Burra, Stergiopoulos, & Rourke, 2009). Caregiver support is usually needed, and public guardianship may be needed in some cases.

Culturally appropriate care involves both addressing the needs of minority ethnocultural groups and addressing the subcultures among elderly people. In general, cultural minorities have less access to mental health services and tend to receive poorer quality care (US Department of Health and Human Services, 2001); thus, building culturally humble and responsive services is critical (Abramson, Trejo, & Lai, 2002). Stigma associated with mental health care both in the older population and in providers is also a barrier to care. Klap, Unroe, and Unützer (2003) noted that significantly fewer older adults with mental illness perceived a need for mental health services compared to younger adults with mental illness. Fewer older adults reported that their primary care physicians asked about anxiety, spent time asking about or addressing mental health issues, or referred them to mental health treatment. This highlights the widespread need for psychoeducation concerning elder mental health.

Medicare, the primary source of health care financing for adults aged 65 years or older in the United States, presents both solutions and challenges for access to care in this population. This entitlement program, created in 1965, is available to all US citizens and most legal permanent residents. In general, Medicare has broad coverage, including coverage of transportation to appointments, home health aides, and day programs, all of which address access to care issues. Seniors who meet income limits are also able to obtain Medicaid. These "dually eligible" individuals can use Medicaid to help pay for premiums and out-of-pocket expenses. Medicaid also covers some services beyond those covered by Medicare, including prescription drugs, eyeglasses, hearing aids, and nursing facility care beyond the 100-day limit ("Seniors & Medicare and Medicaid Enrollees," 2016). However, having to "spend down" assets in order to be able to obtain Medicaid-covered services can be confusing, financially destabilizing, and a barrier to care for many elderly people.

Care coordination for mentally ill older adults plays a crucial role in helping this population navigate a complex and often disjointed system. Draper and Low (2004) reviewed the literature searching for characteristics of effective models of care for older adults. They found that evidence supported the effectiveness of case management, multidisciplinary team-based community services, primary care/specialist care collaborations (for depression), and integrated mental health services. Case management programs can identify patient needs for community-based services and provide linkage to services, as well as advocacy and monitoring.

Building specific, elder-friendly mental health care programs requires a multidimensional partnership among a diverse group of stakeholders. It is increasingly necessary as the demographic reality of the aging population continues to assert itself.

## REFERENCES

Abramson, T. A., Trejo, L., & Lai, D. W. L. (2002). Culture and mental health: Providing appropriate services for a diverse older population. *Generations, 26,* 21–27.

Adelman, R. D., Tmanova, L. L., Delgado, D., Dion, S., & Lachs, M. S. (2014). Caregiver burden: A clinical review. *JAMA, 311*(10), 1052–1060.

Bartels, S. J. (2003). Improving the system of care for older adults with mental illness in the United States: Findings and recommendations for the President's New Freedom Commission on Mental Health. *American Journal of Geriatric Psychiatry, 11*(5), 486–497.

Brookmeyer, R., Johnson, E., Ziegler-Graham, K., & Arrighi, H. M. (2007). Forecasting the global burden of Alzheimer's disease. *Alzheimer's & Dementia, 3*(3), 186–191.

Burra, T. A., Stergiopoulos, V., & Rourke, S. B. (2009). A systematic review of cognitive deficits in homeless adults: Implications for service delivery. *Canadian Journal of Psychiatry, 54*(2), 123–133.

Chun, A. (Ed.). (2011). *Geriatric care by design: A clinician's handbook to meet the needs of older adults through environmental and practice redesign.* New York, NY: American Medical Association.

Cohen, C. I., & Ibrahim, F. (2012). Serving elders in the public sector. In H. L. McQuistion, W. E. Sowers, J. M. Ranz, & J. M. Feldman (Eds.), *Handbook of community psychiatry* (pp. 485–502). New York, NY: Springer.

Draper, B., & Low, L. (2004). *What is the effectiveness of old-age mental health services?* (Health Evidence Network report). Copenhagen, Denmark: World Health Organization Regional Office for Europe. Retrieved from http://www.euro.who.int/document/E83685.pdf. Accessed April 19, 2016.

Faustman, W. O., Moses, J. A., Jr., & Csernansky, J. G. (1990). Limitations of the Mini-Mental State Examination in predicting neuropsychological functioning in a psychiatric sample. *Acta Psychiatrica Scandinavica, 81*(2), 126–131.

Gonyea, J. G., Mills-Dick, K., & Bachman, S. S. (2010). The complexities of elder homelessness, a shifting political landscape and emerging community responses. *Journal of Gerontological Social Work, 53*(7), 575–590.

Green, M. F. (2006). Cognitive impairment and functional outcome in schizophrenia and bipolar disorder. *Journal of Clinical Psychiatry, 67*(10), e12.

Horgan, S., LeClair, K., Donnelly, M., Hinton, G., MacCourt, P., & Krieger-Frost, S. (2009). Developing a national consensus on the accessibility needs of older adults with concurrent and chronic, mental and physical health issues: A preliminary framework informing collaborative mental health care planning. *Canadian Journal on Aging, 28*(2), 97–105.

Institute of Medicine. (2012). *The mental health and substance use workforce for older adults: In whose hands?* Washington, DC: National Academies Press.

Johannesen, M., & LoGiudice, D. (2013). Elder abuse: A systematic review of risk factors in community-dwelling elders. *Age and Ageing, 42*(3), 292–298.

Karp, F. (Ed.). (2011). *Talking with your older patient: A clinician's handbook*. Washington, DC: US Department of Health and Human Services, National Institutes of Health, National Institute on Aging.

Klap, R., Unroe, K. T., & Unützer, J. (2003). Caring for mental illness in the United States: A focus on older adults. *American Journal of Geriatric Psychiatry, 11*(5), 517–524.

Lachs, M. S., & Pillemer, K. A. (2015). Elder abuse. *New England Journal of Medicine, 373*(20), 1947–1956.

Mackin, R. S., & Areán, P. A. (2009). Incidence and documentation of cognitive impairment among older adults with severe mental illness in a community mental health setting. *American Journal of Geriatric Psychiatry, 17*(1), 75–82.

Morley, J. E., Morris, J. C., Berg-Weger, M., Borson, S., Carpenter, B. D., Del Campo, N., . . . Vellas, B. (2015). Brain health: The importance of recognizing cognitive impairment: An IAGG consensus conference. *Journal of the American Medical Directors Association, 16*(9), 731–739.

National Coalition for the Homeless. (2009) *Homelessness among elderly persons*. Retrieved from http://www.nationalhomeless.org/factsheets/Elderly.pdf. Accessed April 19, 2016.

Palinkas, L. A., Criado, V., Fuentes, D., Shepherd, S., Milian, H., Folsom, D., & Jeste, D. V. (2007). Unmet needs for services for older adults with mental illness: Comparison of views of different stakeholder groups. *American Journal of Geriatric Psychiatry, 15*(6), 530–540.

*Seniors & Medicare and Medicaid enrollees*. (2016). Retrieved from https://www.medicaid.gov/medicaid/eligibility/medicaid-enrollees/index.html

US Census Bureau. (2014). *Projections of the population by sex and selected age groups for the United States: 2015 to 2060*. Retrieved from https://www.census.gov/population/projections/data/national/2014/summarytables.html

US Department of Health and Human Services. (2001) *Mental health: Culture, race, and ethnicity—A supplement to mental health: A report of the Surgeon General.* Rockville, MD: US Department of Health and Human Services, Substance Abuse and Mental Health Services Administration, Center for Mental Health Services.

Wolff, J. L., Spillman, B. C., Freedman, V. A., & Kasper, J. D. (2016). A national profile of family and unpaid caregivers who assist older adults with health care activities. *JAMA Internal Medicine, 176*(3), 372–379.

# 15

# Families

**YU-HENG GUO AND ALISON M. HERU** ■

## CASE HISTORY

Mr. Lee, a 30-year-old man with a long history of recurrent major depressive episodes, presents to your clinic seeking treatment for persistent depression, social anxiety, and chronic pain. He first became depressed after his family moved in middle school. He recovered well and went to graduate school, but recurrent depressive episodes prevent him from graduating or maintaining a job. He has been living with his parents since graduation. He has had several adequate medication trials, with limited symptom relief. He attends both individual and group psychotherapy. He has never been hospitalized for psychiatric reasons and does not have a history of suicide attempts.

Mr. Lee's current functioning is poor. He has difficulty with self-care, and spends most of his day isolating. He is afraid to go outside in case he "has to make small talk" or is in pain. His parents tell him "this is all in [his] head" and "they don't understand how [he] can be sick for this long." He reports that his parents make him feel guilty because "they work all day and come home and have to take care of [him]." Mr. Lee's mother drives him to his appointments, and with Mr. Lee's consent, his mother is included in an interview early on. Both parents have given up their hobbies to help out. His father no longer goes to the gym before work so that he can ensure that Mr. Lee takes his morning medications. His mother has to leave work early to drive Mr. Lee to his appointments. Although it is clear that Mr. Lee's mother wants to be helpful, she is quick to tears. She acknowledges that she has been feeling exhausted and has stopped going to church. A family meeting is suggested to bring the whole family unit together, but both mother and patient report they would prefer dealing with their issues individually at this time.

### Clinical Pearl

The impact of mental illness on the family is often overlooked because traditional treatments focus only on the patient. Including the family in appointments is an easy way of gathering data about the patient's support system. In this case, it is clear that the family easily solves practical issues but has difficulty solving emotional problems. When families resist meeting, a more detailed explanation can be given about the goals of a family meeting.

In subsequent meetings, Mr. Lee reports that his depressive symptoms and chronic pain have worsened. He reveals that his brother physically abused him during middle school and high school. He had told his parents about the physical abuse, but he reports that they chalked it up to "playful roughhousing." While in graduate school, he again told his parents about the extent of the abuse. He is angry toward his parents for "not listening" to him, "not protecting" him, and "allowing it to happen." His mood and irritability start to improve as he understands that some of his symptoms function to keep his parents close so that they can protect him. However, he is unable to make any behavioral changes.

Mr. Lee's mother calls you to express frustration with her son's lack of progress. A family meeting is again suggested. You explain that working with the family is an integral part of Mr. Lee's treatment—that a family meeting will help the family determine their roles in treatment and give them an opportunity to ask questions and to better understand the illness. Mr. Lee and his parents agree to a meeting.

### Clinical Pearl

When a patient has been "treatment-resistant" and has failed several adequate trials of antidepressants and psychotherapies, family intervention provides education and support, and it may create the possibility for new solutions. Family intervention may identify dynamics that perpetuate symptoms. Family inclusion can reduce family members' guilt and sadness; address caregiver burden; and support the patient, family, and therapist in working as a team.

During the family meeting, you construct a genogram to better understand the family. You learn that Mr. Lee's older brother had conduct disorder, and although his parents had gotten him into treatment, he was getting bullied at school and his behaviors were difficult to control at home. When Mr. Lee was in middle school, his family moved to a new city and his maternal grandmother passed away. His parents talk about how difficult this time was for the entire family: His mother was grieving and struggling to find a job, his father was working two jobs, and his brother was getting into fights in school.

Mr. Lee identifies with his parents' account and remembers how his mom tried her best to work despite her grief. By acknowledging and mutually engaging in this story, the family begins to create a safe space to discuss difficult feelings and events. It becomes possible to think about how to change the family narrative of hardship.

### Clinical Pearl

A genogram can enrich and give direction on how to change the family narrative. A genogram can include a family history of mental illness and important life events. It can clarify important temporal relationships, such as the life transitions and losses that occurred during the year that Mr. Lee was abused by his brother.

Prior to this meeting, Mr. Lee was so angry at his parents that he forgot that they had been suffering at that time, too. The narrative changed from "my parents did not listen to me and did not protect me" to a narrative about "tragedy within the family and how everyone suffered, despite trying their best."

During the family meeting, Mr. Lee shares his anger with his parents and also acknowledges that they tried their best during difficult times. His parents express guilt about not preventing his brother from hurting him and fear that somehow they "caused" his depression. They recognize that they have overcompensated by "coddling" him and not giving him the space to make progress on his own. This conversation leads Mr. Lee to ask his parents to let him do certain things on his own, such as driving to appointments and taking his medications. He gives them permission to say "This is what we agreed on" if he asks for their help in these situations. House chores and searching for jobs are a difficult negotiation. Mr. Lee expresses that the way in which they ask him about these topics ("Did you do the chores?" and "Did you find a job yet?") makes him feel pressured, overwhelmed, and more avoidant. He suggests that they ask, "How is the job search going? Is there anything I can help you with?" His parents agree.

The family learns about the recurrent nature of his illness and about the roles of medications and different providers. The parents feel less burdened with the responsibility of "making everything better," and they understand that their role in treatment is to be supportive without being "pushy." The family is commended on their strength in discussing these difficult topics and their commitment to helping each other. They have additional questions, such as "How do we talk about his illness with other family members?" and "How do we know when he is doing poorly and we need to intervene?" These are common family questions, and the family is referred to a multifamily psychoeducational group. In this setting, the family learns from professionals and from the experience of other families.

### Clinical Pearl

People with mental illness often fall into the role of the "identified patient" in the family. Having the patient in the "sick role" can serve a purpose (e.g., when there is unresolved guilt in the family). Bringing the family together creates a safe space to identify difficult issues, improve communication, and develop a new family narrative.

In this case, the new narrative is no longer about "abandonment and not being protected." Instead, it is about how the family went through a tragedy together and is still trying to determine how to deal with the aftermath. This shifts the attention away from the "identified patient," which perpetuated Mr. Lee's sick role, and the focus becomes how the family can work better together.

During the next few months, Mr. Lee makes behavioral progress. He takes more ownership of his own mental and physical health, such as eating healthier, exercising, and taking his medications. He drives to his appointments. Although his chronic pain recurs sporadically, his parents are able to support him through these episodes without regression into the sick role. In these instances, they ask him if there is anything they can do to make him more comfortable, but they still expect him to make it to his appointments on his own. Now that his parents know that he wants to hold himself accountable for his medical care, his mother returns to church and his father returns to the gym. The family also sets aside one night a week to go to a movie together.

### Clinical Pearl

The family meeting allows each family member to be open and vulnerable and also to discuss difficult emotions. In this case, this experience translated into more effective communication at home. Clarifying roles helps family members to feel less guilty and to be less reactive, and instead to perform agreed-upon supportive functions. Multifamily psychoeducational groups validate their struggles, help them feel less isolated, and help them improve their coping skills.

Mr. Lee now works as a pharmacy technician. He has tapered off some of his medications. He sees his psychiatrist weekly for individual psychotherapy. The family completed a course of multifamily psychoeducational groups and returned for a second course. They found that they could help other families and enjoyed this experience. Mr. Lee and his parents come for a family session every 4 months.

## DISCUSSION

Research supports family-centered care in psychiatry (Heru, 2015). Family interventions are included in the American Psychiatric Association (APA) practice guidelines for schizophrenia, bipolar disorder, and depression (Heru, 2006). Two simple interventions, family inclusion and family psychoeducation, are well accepted by patients when the purpose is clearly explained and boundaries between individual treatment and family involvement are drawn. Clarifying that the term "family" encompasses supportive friends and community members allows patients who are cut off from families to strengthen their support network.

Engaging families requires positive welcoming statements that affirm that family members are valued and can make important contributions to each other's well-being. Families may need a professional's permission and guidance to carry out supportive functions. Patients also need to know when they should be doing things for themselves and when they can rely on family members. The discussion with the patient regarding family contact must be strong, supportive, and collaborative.

Family inclusion means that the family is simply present during appointments. This can occur as part of routine care. Regardless of the diagnosis, when the family is included in the assessment, decision-making, and treatment planning, patient adherence improves (DiMatteo, 2004). Observing family interactions also helps determine family needs. These needs can be addressed with practical problem-solving, which might include getting medications from the pharmacy or arranging child care. Families that are not able to identify and solve practical problems may also have difficulty identifying or solving emotional problems. Families that show significant conflict, overt disagreement about how to manage the illness, or have family problems that predate the illness will benefit from more intensive family intervention, such as family psychoeducation or family systems consultation.

In addition to providing information about the illness, psychoeducational interventions provide family members with the opportunity to express their feelings and discuss their difficulties managing the illness. Family psychoeducation can be structured as a series of single or multifamily meetings. Multifamily psychoeducational group treatment allows families to learn from each other, explores the meaning of the illness for each family member, and helps the family develop a repertoire of coping skills (McFarlane, 2002). Multifamily psychoeducational groups are considered the standard of care according to the APA guidelines for treatment of schizophrenia (APA, 2004) and the Schizophrenia Patient Outcomes Research Team (PORT) recommendations for the treatment of schizophrenia (Dixon et al., 2010). Family interventions for specific disorders are summarized by Keitner, Heru, and Glick (2010), and specific directions for setting up family psychoeducational programs are described in the *Family Psychoeducational Workbook* (http://www.nebhands.nebraska.edu/files/ FamPsy_Workbook.pdf). Family inclusive treatment (FIT), a specific model of family psychoeducation developed at the Family Center for Bipolar Disorder, engages families at the initiation of treatment and during quarterly family visits, providing relapse prevention planning throughout patient care (Miklowitz, 2010).

Family members frequently blame themselves for their relative's illness and experience rejection and stigmatization from others. High expressed emotion (EE), especially the components of critical comments and hostility, is frequently present in families of poorly functioning patients (Brown & Rutter, 1966). High EE is thought to be derived from family members' lack of understanding of the illness and faulty attributions, and psychoeducation is the treatment of choice for managing a family's high EE (Miklowitz, 2004).

Family systems therapy (FST) aims to disrupt dysfunctional family transactions and promote enhanced functioning. Treatment focuses on improving communication; establishing clear family roles and rules; and enhancing problem-solving, emotional expression, and connection. A meta-analysis that identified 34 studies showed FST to be efficacious for the treatment of mood disorders, eating disorders, substance use disorders, mental and social factors related to medical conditions and physical disorders, and schizophrenia (Von Sydow, Beher, Schweitzer, & Retzlaff, 2010).

Many types of FST, such as structural or strategic family therapy, have been developed since the 1950s. However, in this chapter, as in many clinical situations, we recommend more basic family interventions, such as family inclusion and family psychoeducation, both of which have a substantial evidence base for efficacy (Heru, 2015). Compared to FST, which requires 1 or 2 years of supervised training, family inclusion requires minimal training, and family psychoeducation can be delivered after 4–6 hours of training, using McFarlane's model.

Health care providers may cite concerns about patient confidentiality as a rationale for excluding family members. Guidelines on family-centered care (Heru, 2015; Molinaro, Solomon, Mannion, Cantwell, & Evans, 2012) include obtaining a release to speak with a support person as part of the routine initial paperwork; contacting the support person to discuss key issues; and offering ongoing support, advice, and resources. Family-centered care is normalized by the presence of posters and handouts that describe the evidence that family treatment improves patient outcome. The Association of Family Psychiatrists provides helpful information sheets and websites (http://familypsychiatrists.org). The National Alliance on Mental Illness (NAMI) provides relevant literature and family support. Holding a family day in the clinic for educational programing and social events sends a clear message that families are welcome.

Similar to advanced directives, psychiatric advanced directives (https://www. nami.org) and child and baby care plans (http://www.copmi.net.au/parents-and-families/parents/developing-a-care-plan.html) can be drawn up with patients and their families. These provide physician and health care settings with guidance when patients are temporarily unable to make decisions or are hospitalized.

Public psychiatry sets a strong example for psychiatry by the inclusion of families as members of the treatment team. Knowledgeable families in the community help reduce the substantial burden of mental illness with early identification of symptoms and faster treatment-seeking behavior. Educated families also work in the community to reduce stigma and increase the acceptance of mental health treatment in all settings.

## REFERENCES

American Psychiatric Association Work Group on Schizophrenia. (2004). Practice guideline for the treatment of schizophrenia, 2nd edition. *American Journal of Psychiatry, 161*(2 Suppl.), 1056.

Brown, G. W., & Rutter, M. (1966). The measurement of family activities and relationships: A methodological study. *Human Relations, 19*, 241–258.

DiMatteo, M. (2004). Social support and patient adherence to medical treatment: A meta-analysis. *Health Psychology, 23*, 207–218.

Dixon, L. B., Dickerson, F., Bellack, A. S., Bennett, M., Dickinson, D., Goldberg, R. W., . . . Kreyenbuhl, J.; Schizophrenia Patient Outcomes Research Team (PORT). (2010). The 2009 schizophrenia PORT psychosocial treatment recommendations and summary statements. *Schizophrenia Bulletin, 36*(1), 48–70.

Heru, A. M. (2006). Family psychiatry: From research to practice. *American Journal of Psychiatry, 163*, 962–968.

Heru, A. M. (2015). Family-centered care in the outpatient general psychiatry clinic. *Journal of Psychiatric Practice, 21*(5), 381–388.

Keitner, G. I., Heru, A. M., Glick, I. D. (2010). *Clinical manual of couples and family therapy.* Washington, DC: APPI Press.

McFarlane, W. R. (Ed.). (2002). *Multifamily group treatment for severe psychiatric disorders.* New York, NY: Guilford.

Miklowitz, D. J. (2004). The role of family systems in severe and recurrent psychiatric disorders: A developmental psychopathology view. *Development and Psychopathology, 16*(3), 667–688.

Miklowitz, D. J. (2010). *Bipolar disorder: A family-focused treatment approach* (2nd ed.). New York, NY: Guilford.

Molinaro, M., Solomon, P., Mannion, E., Cantwell, K., & Evans, A. C., Jr. (2012). Development and implementation of family involvement standards for behavioral health provider programs. *American Journal of Psychiatric Rehabilitation, 15*(91), 81–96.

Von Sydow, K., Beher, S., Schweitzer, J., & Retzlaff, R. (2010). The efficacy of systemic therapy with adult patients: A meta-content analysis of 38 randomized controlled trials. *Family Process, 49*(4), 457–485.

# Special Populations

# 16

# State Psychiatric Hospitals

MARY BARBER, FLAVIO CASOY, AND RACHEL ZINNS ■

## CASE HISTORIES

### Case 1

Gracie is a 35-year-old woman with an IQ in the borderline range and a significant trauma history. Her parents both had schizophrenia and alcohol use disorder. She was placed in foster care at an early age, and she suffered physical and sexual trauma over multiple years in different placements, including children's residential placement. From age 15 to the present, she has been in and out of your state hospital, usually for cutting herself or banging her head or for attacking another person. Her current hospital admission is for threatening another woman at her residence with a broken bottle in a dispute over a man in whom they were both interested.

Gracie has been discharged to the state hospital on-campus residence several times in the past few years, but she always returns after another altercation or incident of self-harm. The longest she has been able to remain out of the hospital has been 9 months. Once she is hospitalized, it is often difficult to get her ready to be discharged again because she cuts herself and hits other patients while in the hospital. She often becomes embroiled in drama with the other female patients, sometimes overtly competing to be the most "unstable" patient or becoming jealous of other patients who are leaving the hospital. As soon as discharge is mentioned to her in treatment planning meetings, she seems to regress, reverting to head-banging, throwing things on the unit, and scratching herself.

### Clinical Pearl

This is a familiar scenario in state hospitals—a patient who remains in the hospital because she cannot manage her behavior in the community. Once in the hospital, patients such as Gracie may regress further, sometimes even finding new ways to harm themselves. Often, patients such as Gracie have extensive experience with institutions such as foster care, children's residential settings, hospitals, jails, and prisons. Although they are familiar with institutions, they have experienced them as traumatic and generally do poorly with the conditions created by being in the hospital—being in close contact with other patients, having to abide by unit rules, having to vie for staff attention, lacking freedom of movement, and not having clear positive goals other than the goal of discharge. Helping patients like Gracie to consider and pursue the possibility of recovery is a challenge.

Gracie hit a low point when her best friend on the unit was discharged to an apartment off the hospital campus. She began swallowing objects such as her toothbrush and plastic utensils, necessitating trips to the local hospital for endoscopy. Gracie was put on one-to-one observation and seemed despondent. She became frustrated with her team; accused them of not working hard enough toward her discharge; and had a few episodes of mild physical aggression toward staff, such as spitting and shoving. These behaviors were most acute at change of shift when she knew staff members were going to leave. She would demand to spend time with them as they were walking out the door. She reported feeling abandoned and neglected, while the staff felt frustrated, angry, and helpless.

Her team made a plan to focus on Gracie's strengths and to capitalize on even brief periods without self-harming or violent behaviors. They carefully explained the proposed plan to Gracie, and all agreed that they would not let setbacks derail this plan. For each day Gracie was able to remain safe, she had a reward centered on increasing her freedom. She went on escorted walks around the hospital and trips to the outpatient clubhouse model program on the grounds. Her groups in the hospital were focused on building positive coping strategies and recognizing triggers to self-harm. As she gained confidence, Gracie began to go on day passes to the clubhouse program, where she enjoyed going out with program members to volunteer at a local food and clothing pantry. She reported feeling grateful for the opportunity to help others. Gracie continued to have outbursts at times and swallowed buttons on the weekend after another friend was discharged from the hospital. After these episodes, the team reassured her, paused her passes and privileges briefly, and then returned to the plan. At this point, Gracie is actively planning for discharge from the hospital. Staff report feeling hopeful for Gracie and invested in her growing independence, and they enjoy chatting with her during meals and other unstructured times.

### Clinical Pearl

In the community, patients such as Gracie bounce between short-stay acute hospitals, jails, psychiatric emergency rooms, and shelters because of their extreme behaviors. State hospitals often have an array of services on the same campus that can be selected and organized to provide support for these types of patients. In addition to locked, secure units with psychiatrists and nurses, state hospitals often have a robust rehabilitation department and the ability to provide psychosocial programming that insurance generally does not reimburse in acute care hospitals. In addition, on campus there are often unlocked residences with 24-hour staffing, an outpatient clinic serving both patients living in the residences and patients from the surrounding community, and a clubhouse where patients can socialize and develop independence and leadership skills.

Patients with significant childhood trauma, abandonment, and developmental delay pose a major challenge to community organizations because of their volatility and intensity of need for staff time and attention. In a state hospital, patients such as Gracie are at significant risk of regressing and losing independent living skills, but there is time and opportunity for staff to develop healing relationships with patients and help patients transition at their own pace.

## Case 2

Martin is a 32-year-old man with schizophrenia. He has been receiving services from the state hospital clinic in his neighborhood for the past year. In early adulthood, he was in and out of local hospitals due to auditory hallucinations and the belief that he was being influenced by "demons." At times he was suicidal, and in one incident he attacked his sister with a knife, thinking she was part of an evil conspiracy. During these years of illness, Martin dropped out of college, where he had been studying fine art, and he was unable to keep any job for more than a few weeks.

After many shorter term hospital stays, he was referred to the state hospital, where he was kept for 4 months. During that time, he was started and stabilized on clozapine. He also received cognitive remediation treatment in a group setting led by psychologists. Martin describes that when he got to a certain dose of clozapine, his hallucinations and suicidal thoughts "went away completely" and have not returned since. He was discharged to a supported apartment program with a case manager who visits him weekly. He sees his therapist weekly at the state-run clinic and has monthly appointments with his psychiatrist.

While Martin was still an inpatient, he began attending art therapy groups. This was the beginning of his return to painting and photography, which he had left behind during his earlier period of illness. The vocational counselor in the hospital worked with Martin on a goal of returning to college. By the time he was discharged from the hospital, Martin had had a small art show at the library close to the hospital, and he was beginning to take art classes again at the local community college. Now 1 year later, he is exhibiting his work regularly, working part-time at an art supply store, and continuing to take classes toward his degree.

### Clinical Pearl

The luxury of time can help someone with serious mental illness make significant steps toward recovery during a hospital stay. One could argue that Martin might have achieved a similar outcome if he had coordinated outpatient treatment that offered clozapine, integrated vocational services, and cognitive remediation. This type of integrated treatment is evidence based (Kane et al., 2015) (Olfson, Gerhard, Crystal, & Stroup, 2016), but many patients are not able to get such high-quality treatment in the community.

## DISCUSSION

State psychiatric hospitals treat people with the most complex serious mental illnesses. They are the specialty medical centers for psychiatric illness. Traditionally, the general public and even mental health professionals hold the image of state hospitals as places for long-term housing and custodial care (Litvak, 1948; Payne, 2009).

In fact, today's state hospitals emphasize active treatment, with the goal of returning patients to the community once they no longer need inpatient care. State hospitals frequently operate not only inpatient beds but also a system that includes clinics, assertive community treatment teams, clubhouses and other rehabilitation programs, as well as outpatient residences. This in-house continuum of care can support a coordinated transition from a long inpatient stay back into the community.

State hospitals do not bill for the majority of inpatient services. This creates both freedom and constraint for the state hospital system. On the one hand, state services are viewed as total cost centers in the state budget and are not credited for any revenues. As such, state services are vulnerable to budget cuts. On the other hand, state services do not have the constant pressure that other mental health systems of care experience—to make revenue targets, to cut services that do not produce billing, and to plan services with an eye toward fiscal viability. Although state hospital administrators have in mind the cost of daily hospitalization, they are not beholden to an insurance company to keep length of stay to a certain number of days.

In the United States, outpatient services are often fragmented, and services such as rehabilitation are threatened by low reimbursement. Acute psychiatric inpatient units have gone to what some have described as "ultrashort" lengths of stay, in which goals must be extremely limited and focused on rapid stabilization (Glick, Sharfstein, & Schwartz, 2011). In this environment, state hospitals are often the only place where meaningful inpatient treatment can occur and where a complex illness can be treated in an interdisciplinary manner using a network of care.

State hospitals have their downside as well. When patients stay for extended periods in the hospital, they may become overly acculturated to the hospital structure or "institutionalized." They can develop routinized and maladaptive patterns of interacting with staff that have nothing to do with psychosis but that lead staff and outside providers to assess, for example, "He is too ill for the community." Patients lose their ability to problem-solve and care for themselves, and they lose connections with the outside community that would allow them to successfully transition out of the hospital. In the face of numerous rejections by outside agencies, staff members lose hope that their work will result in the patient's discharge. Clinicians and administrators who work in these settings must continually develop programming to help patients advance their self-management skills, and they must support staff in working persistently with patients to help them transition out of restrictive settings. The 1999 Olmstead lawsuit, involving disabled adults who were unable to move on from an adult home, ended in a decision asserting that patients must be placed in the least restrictive setting. This decision has made helping patients move out of the hospital and into more independent settings even more pressing.

The state hospital was once the centerpiece of care for serious mental illness. In the 1960s, deinstitutionalization began in response to many factors—overcrowded hospitals, state budget cuts, and importantly, the introduction of antipsychotic medications. Funding poured into community services as state hospital patients were discharged, but much of that funding was used for treatment tailored to independently functioning patients rather than those with serious mental illness. Reinvestment funding followed in many waves to try to target resources to the neediest patients. Even so, advocates have argued that as the state hospital system has shrunk, community services have never been built up proportionately. Some point to problems such as the homeless mentally ill as a result of this imbalance.

A disproportionate number of people with serious mental illness are institutionalized in prisons (Lamb & Weinberger, 1998).

State hospitals continue to be under threat: The number of beds has continued to shrink each year since deinstitutionalization began in the 1960s (Fisher, Geller, & Pandiani, 2009; Parks & Radke, 2014). From 1997 to 2015, the number of state psychiatric hospitals in the United States declined from 254 to 195 (24% decrease), and the number of beds decreased by 39% during the same period (NRI, 2015). Twenty-four states have just one or two state psychiatric hospitals—states with only one hospital include Vermont, New Hampshire, Utah, New Mexico, and Arizona (NRI, 2015). State hospital beds have continued to be subject to cuts as state budgets become leaner. For example, Rockland Psychiatric Center in New York's Hudson Valley once had 9,000 inpatients living on its grounds. Today, the hospital has 370 inpatients, and three other state hospitals in the area have closed in the past 20 years.

Today, in most states, an increasing portion of state inpatient beds are reserved for people with forensic histories who are referred through jails and prisons (Fisher et al., 2009; Parks & Radke, 2014). In some states, virtually all the remaining state beds are for forensic patients.

The two cases discussed in this chapter illustrate how state hospitals can play a positive role in the treatment of patients with serious mental illness. Many patients, like Gracie and Martin, have been rejected by other providers or never were able to be effectively treated until they came into contact with state hospital services. State hospitals' freedom from constraints of discharge pressure and the need to generate revenues means they have resources that the rest of the public system can generally no longer afford. Whether the system can be allowed to shrink further and yet still be accessible to patients who need it is currently a subject of debate.

## REFERENCES

Fisher, W. H., Geller, J. L., & Pandiani, J. A. (2009). The changing role of the state psychiatric hospital. *Health Affairs*, *28*(3), 676–684.

Glick, I. D., Sharfstein, S. S., & Schwartz, H. I. (2011). Inpatient psychiatric care in the 21st century: The need for reform. *Psychiatric Services*, *62*(2), 206–209.

Kane, J. M., Robinson, D. G., Schooler, N. R., Mueser, K. T., Penn, D. L., Rosenheck, R. A., . . . Heinssen, R. K. (2015). Comprehensive versus usual community care for first-episode psychosis: 2-year outcomes from the NIMH RAISE early treatment program. *American Journal of Psychiatry*, *173*(4), 362–372.

Lamb, H. R., & Weinberger, L. E. (1998). Persons with mental illness in jails and prisons: A review. *Psychiatric Services*, *49*(4),483–492.

Litvak, A. (1948). *The snake pit*. 20th Century Fox Films.

NRI. (2015). *Tracking the history of state psychiatric hospital closures from 1997 to 2015*. Falls Church, VA: Author. Retrieved from https://www.nri-inc.org

Olfson, M., Gerhard, T., Crystal, S., & Stroup, T. S. (2016). Clozapine for schizophrenia: State variation in evidence-based practice. *Psychiatric Services*, *67*(2), 152.

Parks, J., & Radke, A. Q. (2014). *The vital role of state psychiatric hospitals*. Alexandria, VA: National Association of State Mental Health Program Directors.

Payne, C. (2009). *Asylum: Inside the closed world of state mental hospitals*. Cambridge, MA: MIT Press.

# 17

# Forensic Psychiatry

**SHEKU MAGONA AND TARA STRAKA** ∎

## CASE HISTORY

Robert is a 34-year-old single, homeless, unemployed African American man charged with attempted burglary in the second degree with a maximum sentence of 7 years. He is admitted to a state forensic psychiatric hospital for fitness restoration after having been detained in a city jail for 3 months. He was arrested after police were called by an apartment building resident who thought the defendant appeared to want to gain entrance to the ground-floor apartments as he reportedly was observed pushing and pulling on doorknobs. As per police reports, he had no authority, permission, or legal reason to be present in the building. At the time of arrest, the defendant was reportedly disorderly and was found to be in possession of a small amount of cannabis. He informed the arresting officers that he was trying to keep warm.

### Clinical Pearl

The most common reason for defendants to be found unfit to proceed with their criminal cases is psychosis (Bertman et al., 2003). Patients admitted to forensic hospitals for treatment to restore competency commonly carry primary psychotic diagnoses, including schizophrenia, schizoaffective disorder, and bipolar disorder. Other symptoms of mental illness that can interfere with fitness include mania, severe depression, and affective dysregulation associated with personality disorders.

Robert had been homeless for the prior 9 months after leaving a residential treatment facility. He was previously taking oral risperidone and benztropine. The residence reports he was suspected of using drugs and failed a urine test, so the residence discussed with him possible changes in his privileges. This news led to Robert walking away from the residence. He reports sleeping in parks, church entrances, and on church pews, as well as using the subway for the winter. He gave no clear reason why he did not go to a shelter or consider returning to the residence. He is estranged from a religiously observant parent and two older male siblings because of his psychiatric illness and cannabis use.

When Robert was arrested and brought to jail, he was found to be self-isolating and not eating, and he was subsequently relocated to the mental observation unit. He was described as intermittently compliant with prescribed medications. He was taken to a city hospital inpatient forensic ward for fitness evaluations on three occasions, but he refused to cooperate with his lawyer or evaluators. Robert gave little reason for his refusal to cooperate in the first meeting, and during the second, he voiced distrust of the court-appointed lawyer. Two fitness evaluators, a psychiatrist and a psychologist at the mental health court clinic, found Robert incompetent to stand trial and recommended longitudinal observation and inpatient competency restoration.

## Clinical Pearl

Having mental illness alone does not predict or determine that a defendant will be incompetent. *Dusky v. United States* was a 1960 Supreme Court case that outlined the basic legal standard for determining competency and affirmed a defendant's right to have a competency evaluation before proceeding to trial. The Court ruled in the *Dusky* decision (as cited in Rosner, 2003) that to be fit to proceed, a defendant must have "sufficient present ability to consult with his lawyer with a reasonable degree of rational understanding" and a "rational as well as factual understanding of the proceedings against him" (p. 187). This case set a federal standard for competency that is used nationwide to determine if a defendant is fit to proceed to trial, as well as to plead guilty or to waive the right to counsel. If a defendant is declared by the court (with the help of forensic expert psychiatrists and psychologists) as incompetent, criminal and judicial proceedings are put on hold until the defendant's deficits are addressed and competency is restored. Such a process can dramatically lengthen the time from arrest to disposition for these mentally ill defendants.

Robert's first psychiatric hospitalization was at age 19 years when he was in college. He was hospitalized for 6 weeks after several months of falling grades, poor self-care, and increased self-isolation. He had become threatening toward his then roommate. He has received social security disability benefits for a diagnosis of schizophrenia; he has no other medical conditions. A review of past records with the help of his lawyer reveals six prior inpatient psychiatric hospitalizations, including one 4-month hospitalization 8 years ago in a state psychiatric hospital after he was found incompetent to stand trial on misdemeanor charges of trespassing. He required a treatment over objection court order to restore him to competency.

## Clinical Pearl

Treatment over objection is a common component of fitness restoration treatment, because impaired insight is a frequent clinical problem for these patients. There is no national standard for the process of treatment over objection. The courts have recognized that involuntary treatment with psychiatric medication is a deprivation of civil liberties and, therefore, requires due process. However, that process varies state by state and may involve administrative or judicial review.

It is not uncommon for a defendant to be readmitted multiple times to a forensic hospital for treatment because he or she stops adhering to medication after returning to jail following fitness restoration. This "revolving door" can substantially lengthen the time to disposition of the legal case and the time the defendant is in custody. Long-acting antipsychotic medications can help patients remain clinically stable for longer periods after returning to jail—ideally long enough to have their cases disposed.

On examination, Robert is a tall, disheveled man of slim build with limited eye contact. His speech is difficult to understand at times, because his volume is low and tapers off. His thought process is disorganized with possible thought blocking—the interviewers had to repeat questions. He denies suicidal or homicidal ideation. He does not endorse perceptual disturbances but at times appears internally preoccupied. His mood is described as "fine"; his affect is restricted but became irritable when charges came up in discussion. Robert has limited insight and judgment with regard to his illness, the need for continued treatment, and his legal options. He demonstrates adequate impulse control. He is alert and oriented to person, place, time, and events. He was able to do calculations and has fair remote, recent, and immediate memory.

A treatment over objection application was granted for the long-acting form of risperidone, and Robert was restored to fitness. The forensic psychiatrist who oversaw his restoration advocated to the judge that Robert be referred to a community-based diversion program with an assertive community treatment (ACT) team. Robert demonstrated that he understood the need to adhere to the conditions of the diversion. Although he returned to a shelter initially, the ACT team was eventually able to help him secure supported housing. He also began vocational training. Two years later, he is still working with the ACT team and has not been arrested again.

## Clinical Pearl

The terms *diversion* and *alternatives to incarceration* refer to programs that divert people with serious mental illness and often co-occurring substance use disorders away from jail and provide linkages to support services and community-based treatment. Appropriate diversion may benefit not only the mentally ill individual but also the criminal justice system and the community. Diversion programs reduce frequency and length of incarceration, recidivism, substance use, and the number of psychiatric hospitalizations over the long term (Ryan, Brown, & Watanabe-Galloway, 2010). These programs also may decrease homelessness and improve work stability and community adjustment (Ryan et al., 2010). Robert will be a good candidate for diversion, given his response to treatment, minimal past interaction with the criminal justice system, and willingness to engage with support services. It was important that his forensic psychiatrists had a community psychiatry perspective and could recognize and address the root causes of his recidivism, which included homelessness and a subsequent lack of engagement with treatment. Their advocacy prevented Robert from needing to serve a long prison sentence.

## DISCUSSION

### Background

The mentally ill are overrepresented in US jails and prisons, and as Ryan et al. (2010, p. 470) noted, "the absolute number of persons with severe mental illness is greater in American jails and prisons than in our hospitals, making jails the largest de facto institution for the mentally ill population" (p. 470). In addition to the process of deinstitutionalization that occurred in the United States in the 1960s and 1970s, there are several factors that contribute to the criminalization of the mentally ill (Osher, 2012). Poor access to community services means at-risk individuals remain untreated in the community and, as a result, are more likely to be arrested. The mentally ill are also at increased risk of developing a substance use disorder, and incarceration rates are higher for individuals with co-occurring disorders. Mentally ill defendants are more likely to have been homeless at the time of their arrest, leading to their difficulties being more visible in the community and more likely to draw calls to law enforcement. Once in jail, people with mental illness tend to stay longer and are less likely to successfully achieve probation or parole compared to their non-mentally ill counterparts. Once released, without adequate treatment and social supports, mentally ill individuals are more likely to recidivate. Note, however, that contrary to popular belief, most people with mental illness are not violent, and most people who commit violent crimes are not mentally ill. The mentally ill are far more likely to be victims rather than perpetrators of crime (Osher, 2012).

### Fitness Restoration

Most defendants are restored to fitness; the restorability rate varies from 75% to 90% (Mossman, 2007), depending on the nature and severity of the illness (Kaufman, Way, & Suardi, 2012; Rodol, Epson, & Bloom, 2013). It is usually difficult to predict who can be restored to fitness. However, people with treatment refractory psychotic disorders or developmental, cognitive, or dementing disorders are generally viewed as not restorable (Advokat, Guidry, Burnett, Manguno-Mire, & Thompson, 2012; Morris & Parker, 2009).

Treatment refractory patients who cannot be restored to fitness pose a particular challenge. Prior to the 1972 Supreme Court ruling in *Jackson v. Indiana*, there was no statute of limitations on how long an incompetent defendant could be held for treatment. In this case, the Court (as cited in Rosner, 2003) determined that

> a person charged by a State with a criminal offense who is committed solely on account of his incapacity to proceed to trial cannot be held more than the reasonable period of time necessary to determine whether there is a substantial probability that he will attain that capacity in the foreseeable future. If it is determined that this is not the case, then the State must either institute the customary civil commitment proceeding that would be required to commit indefinitely any other citizen, or release the defendant. (p. 851)

The Court did not, however, define what constituted a "reasonable period of time." Following this finding, many states have enacted periodic judicial review of defendants who are found incompetent and have limited the retention period so as not to exceed the maximum sentence that a person would have received if convicted on his or her charges.

An expeditious and transparent competency restoration ensures the integrity of the legal process while reassuring the public of the fairness and longevity of the results (Fogel, Schiffman, Mumley, Tillbrook, & Grisso, 2013), and it also avoids lengthy involuntary hospitalization. Most states use traditional psychiatric inpatient units or long-term care facilities to achieve fitness restoration. However, given the cost, some states are now exploring restoration on an accelerated basis in jails (Rice & Jennings, 2014). Antipsychotic and mood-stabilizing medications are mainstays of fitness restoration, because medication treatment is the only intervention closely correlated with restoration.

However, psychotherapy and psychoeducation are also key components of treatment. There is evidence that frequent, individualized legal rights education is an effective best practice strategy (Bertman et al., 2003; Morris & Deyoung, 2012).

## Diversion

Diversion programs have several key functions. They define a target group for services, and they screen and identify individuals as early as possible once they have entered the criminal justice system. They also negotiate community-based treatment alternatives, and they implement linkages to systems of care and community supervision. Effective programs successfully balance the mental health needs of the individual with accountability to the court.

These alternatives to incarceration may be voluntary or involuntary and occur at different points in the criminal justice process. Treatment may be a condition of bail. In other cases, prosecution or sentencing may be deferred for a specified period of time, pending successful program completion, while defendants undergo continuing criminal justice supervision during treatment. In still other cases, mentally ill defendants may plead guilty, with a treatment program as a condition of probation.

The sequential intercept model describes the various points within the criminal justice system at which a mentally ill person may be diverted (Munetz & Griffin, 2006). These intercepts are (1) initial contact with local law enforcement or emergency services, (2) initial court appearance, (3) jail or specialty courts (mental health courts and drug courts), (4) re-entry programs from jails and prison, and (5) community-based monitoring of justice-involved patients through probation or parole boards. Diversion programs can be defined by whether diversion occurs "pre-booking" (intercept 1) or "post-booking."

Pre-booking diversion occurs at the point of initial contact with law enforcement— that is, the encounter with police, before arrest or formal charges. This strategy relies heavily on effective interactions between the police and community mental health services. Most pre-booking programs involve specialized training for police officers. A crucial component to this process is the establishment of a drop-off center that has a no-refusal policy for police cases (Hartford et al., 2006).

Post-booking diversion programs may intervene at various points after arrest, including immediately after booking into jail and before formal filing of charges, upon release from pretrial detention, in the setting of an offer for deferred prosecution, at disposition, at sentencing, or in the context of violation of probation. Post-booking diversion programs use a number of clinical tools, including ACT, intensive case management, and residential support, as well as supervision and monitoring from the criminal justice system through intensive psychiatric probation and parole. Mental health courts also play a role in post-booking diversion. These involve a collaborative team of criminal justice staff and treatment providers who employ a problem-solving approach to optimize a defendant's disposition.

The Nathaniel Project is an alternative to incarceration program for people with serious mental illness who are charged with felony offenses in New York City. This program is a best practice diversion model recognized by the American Psychiatric Association Achievement Award (APA, 2002). The program links mentally ill defendants to treatment and housing, and it provides intensive case management and court advocacy. Defendants are referred to the program before final sentencing, which is deferred while they enter treatment for a 2-year period. Regular reports are made to the courts so that cases may be adjudicated without the defendants serving time in prison. However, defendants who do not meet their treatment plan goals may be arrested and incarcerated. By giving the defendants an opportunity to demonstrate that they can engage in treatment and be successful and law-abiding in the community, the program helps them build a new, more favorable track record. The staff work with defendants to develop insight into the connection between their offending behavior and symptoms of mental illness and also to overcome negative perceptions of mental health treatment. The program has been successful in retaining participants and has demonstrated a decrease in arrest rates. It has received funding from both mental health and criminal justice agencies while also demonstrating that the yearly cost of providing services is significantly less than the cost of a year in prison. The Nathaniel Project has played an important role in promoting dialogue between mental health and criminal justice systems.

As part of a Substance Abuse and Mental Health Services Administration initiative, Steadman et al. (Steadman, Morris, & Dennis, 1995; Steadman et al., 1999) delineated key elements common to the most successful jail diversion programs. *Interagency collaboration* involving mental health, criminal justice, corrections, substance abuse treatment, medical care, housing, and social services, with ongoing *active involvement* with regular meetings for service coordination, is essential. A *strong leader, boundary-spanning staff,* and *cross-trained case managers* who have knowledge and experience with both mental health and criminal justice systems are also crucial.

Defendants with serious mental illness are often viewed as fitting poorly within both criminal justice and traditional mental health settings. They are often denied access to treatment and housing in the community, setting up a cycle of reincarceration. Whether diversion occurs pre- or post-booking, the most effective programs operate from the perspective that defendants are citizens of the community who need access to mental health, substance abuse, and psychosocial services. Clinical and administrative leadership from public psychiatrists is essential for the continued development of integrated models of care that bring together the mental health and criminal justice systems.

## REFERENCES

Advokat, C. D., Guidry, D., Burnett, D. M., Manguno-Mire, G., & Thompson, J. W., Jr. (2012). Competency restoration treatment: Differences between defendants declared competent or incompetent to stand trial. *Journal of the American Academy of Psychiatry and the Law, 40*(1), 89–97.

American Psychiatric Association. (2002). Significant achievement awards: The Nathaniel Project—An effective alternative to incarceration. *Psychiatric Services, 53*(10), 1314–1315.

Bertman, L. J., Thompson, J. W., Waters, W. F., Estupinan-Kane, L., Martin, J. A., & Russell, L. (2003). Effect of an individualized treatment protocol on restoration of competency in pretrial forensic inpatients. *Journal of the American Academy of Psychiatry and the Law, 31*(1), 27–35.

Fogel, M. H., Schiffman, W., Mumley, D., Tillbrook, C., & Grisso, T. (2013). Ten year research update (2001–2010): Evaluations for competence to stand trial (adjudicative competence). *Behavioral Sciences & the Law, 31*(2), 165–191. doi:10.1002/bsl.2051

Hartford, K., Carey, R., & Mendonca, J. (2006). Pre-arrest diversion of people with mental illness: Literature review and international survey. *Behavioral Sciences & the Law, 24*, 845–856.

Kaufman, A. R., Way, B. B., & Suardi, E. (2012). Forty years after Jackson v. Indiana: States' compliance with "reasonable period of time" ruling. *Journal of the American Academy of Psychiatry and the Law, 40*(2), 261–265.

Morris, D. R., & Deyoung, N. J. (2012). Psycholegal abilities and restoration of competence to stand trial. *Behavioral Sciences & the Law, 30*(6), 710–728. doi:10.1002/bsl.2040

Morris, D. R., & Parker, G. F. (2009). Effects of advanced age and dementia on restoration of competence to stand trial. *International Journal of Law & Psychiatry, 32*(3), 156–160. doi:10.1016/j.ijlp.2009.02.009

Mossman, D. (2007). Predicting restorability of incompetent criminal defendants. *Journal of the American Academy of Psychiatry and the Law, 35*(1), 34–43.

Munetz, M. R., & Griffin, P. A. (2006). Use of the sequential intercept model as an approach to decriminalization of people with serious mental illness. *Psychiatric Services, 57*(4), 544–549.

Osher, F. C. (2012). Criminal justice: Promoting public health and public safety. In H. L. McQuistion, W. E. Sowers, J. M. Ranz, & J. M. Feldman. (Eds.), *Handbook of community psychiatry* (pp. 423–434). New York, NY: Springer.

Rice, K., & Jennings, J. L. (2014). The ROC program: Accelerated restoration of competency in a jail setting. *Journal of Correctional Health Care, 20*(1), 59–69. doi:10.1177/1078345813505067

Rodol, L., Epson, M. F., & Bloom, J. D. (2013). Limitations of constitutional protections in Jackson v. Indiana pertaining to charges with no statute of limitations. *Journal of the American Academy of Psychiatry and the Law, 41*(1), 114–120.

Rosner, R. (Ed.). (2003). *Principles and practice of forensic psychiatry* (2nd ed.). Boca Raton, FL: CRC Press.

Ryan, S., Brown, C. B., & Watanabe-Galloway, S. (2010). Toward successful postbooking diversion: What are the next steps? *Psychiatric Services, 61*(5), 469–477.

Steadman, H. J., Deane, M. W., Morrissey, J. P., Westcott, M. L., Salasin, S., & Shapiro, S. (1999). A SAMHSA research initiative assessing the effectiveness of jail diversion programs for mentally ill persons. *Psychiatric Services, 50*(12), 1620–1623.

Steadman, H. J., Morris, S. M., & Dennis, D. L. (1995). The diversion of mentally ill persons from jails to community-based services: A profile of programs. *American Journal of Public Health, 85*(12), 1630–1635.

# 18

# Correctional Settings

ELIZABETH FORD ■

## CASE HISTORY

Mr. Hernandez is a 26-year-old single, Hispanic man who has been in treatment with you in an urban community outpatient clinic for approximately 6 months. He was referred to the clinic following a brief psychiatric hospitalization in the context of progressive irritability and violence toward his girlfriend, difficulty sleeping, panic attacks, thoughts of harming himself, and new episodes of binge drinking resulting in several blackouts. In the hospital, he was diagnosed with substance-induced bipolar disorder and alcohol use disorder, and he was treated with a mood stabilizer. You have been seeing him for monthly psychopharmacology sessions and are collaborating with his therapist, a social worker in your clinic. During the 6 months, and in the context of sobriety, his diagnosis has been refined to bipolar II disorder and alcohol use disorder, moderate.

Mr. Hernandez has been well engaged in his treatment and consistent with his appointments, but he suddenly stops attending his visits with you and his therapist. You call his girlfriend. She tells you that he was arrested for hitting someone on the bus and is now in jail.

### Clinical Pearl

Studies have found that one in four people with mental disorders have histories of arrest and that 1% of all police encounters involve people with mental disorders (Livingston, 2016). Individuals with serious mental illness have a slightly increased risk of personal violence (Flynn, Rodway, Appleby, & Shaw, 2014), exacerbated by substance use, and are at increased risk of reincarceration (Baillargeon, Binswanger, Penn, Williams, & Murray, 2009). They are arrested for violent felonies less frequently than for other offenses (Fisher, Grudzinskas, Roy-Bujnowski, & Wolff, 2011). This is striking when compared with the data that, controlling for charge and demographic variables, mentally ill inmates are more likely than their non-mentally ill counterparts to be victimized in correctional settings, receive "infractions" for rule-breaking, and have longer lengths of stay in custody (Council of State Governments, 2012).

Mr. Hernandez is arrested on a felony assault charge and booked into the local jail, under the control of the city's Department of Correction (DOC). He is placed in a holding pen while he awaits a more permanent housing assignment based on his level of security risk (e.g., gang involvement, prior history in the jail, and violence) and his health needs. He is screened by a correctional officer for suicide risk and by a physician assistant for medical and mental health issues.

## Clinical Pearl

Suicide is the leading single cause of death in US jails (Noonan, Rohloff, & Ginder, 2015); this has been the case since the US Department of Justice began reporting death in custody statistics in 2000. As of 2013, the rate of suicide in jail was 46 per 100,000 inmates, which is more than three times the rate in the general US population. Sixty percent of the individuals committing suicide were aged 25–44 years, with men committing suicide at higher rates than women. Rates of suicide in state prison are lower than those in jail (15 per 100,000 prisoners), and suicide is less frequent than deaths attributable to more chronic conditions such as heart disease, liver disease, cancer, and respiratory disease. This reflects the different populations incarcerated in jails and prisons. Jails are designed as short-stay detention facilities for individuals awaiting trial or for those who are sentenced to less than 1 year. Prisons are designed as long-term facilities for individuals sentenced to more than 1 year and have, on average, older inmates than those in jail.

Mr. Hernandez denies any suicidal thoughts and reports that his last drinking binge was approximately 24 hours ago, leading to a blackout and the behavior that led to his arrest. He denies any psychiatric history but is referred for a mental health appointment for the following week and is started on a benzodiazepine taper to reduce the risk of alcohol withdrawal.

## Clinical Pearl

Substance use disorders are the most frequently diagnosed mental health disorders in correctional settings (American Psychiatric Association [APA] Workgroup, 2015) and are associated with criminal behavior in the community related to using, procuring, or selling the substance (Nunn et al., 2009). The National Commission for Correctional Health Care (NCCHC, 2014), an accrediting agency for jails and prisons that was formed in the 1970s by the American Medical Association, requires that protocols exist in jails for safely managing alcohol/sedative withdrawal. Very few correctional institutions in the United States continue or initiate opioid replacement therapy (ORT) for substance dependence (Nunn et al., 2009); the New York City jail system was the first to do so. State and federal prisons typically do not offer ORT and therefore require an individual to be detoxified, sometimes rapidly, prior to admission.

Mr. Hernandez is housed in a general population housing area with 35 other men with varying degrees of health and mental health issues. He witnesses several fights among his peers, one requiring the DOC staff to use chemical spray to contain the violence. He sleeps only a few hours each night, both afraid for his safety and anxious about what will happen in his legal case. He starts pacing at night and getting into arguments during the day. One of the other inmates steals Mr. Hernandez's phone card so that he can no longer call his girlfriend. On his fifth day in jail, Mr. Hernandez tells the officer watching his housing area that he is thinking of killing himself. The officer brings Mr. Hernandez to the medical clinic, and a psychiatrist sees him. During the session, he says that he can no longer be in his housing area and that he needs to "get out" or else he will hurt himself. He refuses to answer most of the follow-up questions and tells the psychiatrist that she just needs to move him to a different house. He answers "I don't know" to questions about depression and suicidal thinking. Without much history provided and his initial denial of a mental health history, the psychiatrist wonders if Mr. Hernandez is malingering symptoms in order to be moved to a different housing area. She prescribes trazodone for sleep and schedules a follow-up appointment for the next week.

## Clinical Pearl

Without reliable collateral information and clinical history, a definitive mental health diagnosis can be difficult to make. Inmates frequently underreport symptoms in order to avoid associated stigma or overreport in order to obtain alternative housing, avoid punitive segregation (also known as solitary confinement), or impact their criminal case. Because none of the DSM field trials were conducted on prisoners, some of the diagnostic criteria do not match well to the jail or prison setting. In terms of risk to health, underdiagnosis, as in Mr. Hernandez's case, and missing serious illness or risk of injury are a greater concern than overdiagnosis. However, the risk of prescribing medications inappropriately or assigning an incorrect diagnosis of serious mental illness should not be minimized. The DSM-5 (APA, 2013) acknowledges some of these challenges by noting that "under some circumstances, malingering may represent adaptive behavior" and by the addition to "Other Conditions That May Be a Focus of Clinical Attention" of "Problems Related to Crime or Interaction with the Legal System," specifically the V code "Imprisonment or Other Incarceration."

During the next few days, Mr. Hernandez still struggles to sleep and becomes increasingly irritable. He avoids eye contact with his new therapist and stays mostly to himself. He refuses his medication and, one morning, spits on an officer who tells him that he has to wait for a shower. Mr. Hernandez is charged with an infraction, or jail-based crime, and is moved to a punitive segregation, or solitary confinement, unit. After 2 days of being locked in his cell for 23 hours per day, Mr. Hernandez tries to hang himself from an exposed pipe using a torn bed sheet. He is stopped by the officer making rounds and is transferred to the jail-based mental health infirmary for a higher level of care. While in the infirmary, a social worker interviews Mr. Hernandez and identifies his outpatient clinic. She calls the clerk at the clinic for medical records. The clerk replies that she needs a release of information in order to share clinical information; Mr. Hernandez refuses to sign.

## Clinical Pearl

The Health Insurance Portability and Accountability Act of 1996 (HIPAA) is frequently misinterpreted to mean that written authorization is required for any release of protected health information (PHI) in any circumstance. However, there are a number of exceptions for which, according to HIPAA, an authorization or opportunity to agree or object is not required. This includes correctional settings (45 Code of Federal Regulations Subtitle A,164.152, section k(5)):

A covered entity may disclose to a correctional institution or law enforcement officials PHI if information is necessary for the provision of health care, the health and safety of the individual or other inmates, health or safety of officers or employees/law enforcement on the premises of the jail (e.g., maintenance of security), the administration and maintenance of the safety, security and good order of the correctional institution.

Although local laws vary, the intent of this particular federal legislation is to allow for more, not less, sharing of important and often difficult-to-obtain clinical information between community and correctional health care providers. This information exchange is important not only to continue and/or improve clinical care but also to foster the integration of correctional psychiatry into the larger public psychiatry field.

With more clarity about his history, diagnosis, and treatment, Mr. Hernandez is started on a mood stabilizer, encouraged to attend the jail-based Alcoholics Anonymous meetings, and assigned a therapist to meet with him at least once per week. He gives permission for his social worker to contact his public defender, who in turn requests that his criminal case be moved to a specialty mental health court (see Chapter 17). After 4 months, the judge and prosecuting attorney agree to an alternative to incarceration in a dual-diagnosis program affiliated with your outpatient clinic along with monthly psychopharmacology sessions with you.

When he returns to your care, Mr. Hernandez is cautious and reserved. He avoids eye contact, spends much of the session without speaking, and looks tired.

### Clinical Pearl

The experience of incarceration, depending on the length of time, resilience of the individual, and exposure to direct and witnessed trauma either before or during incarceration, can have intense and lasting emotional effects. "Correctional adaptation," "prisonization," or the evolution of attitudes and behaviors that may be adaptive and useful in a correctional environment but problematic in mental health settings (e.g., isolation, manipulation, vigilance, and limited trust) can lead to treatment challenges upon re-entry (Carr et al., 2006). Incarcerated individuals, especially women, have higher prevalence rates of trauma exposure and post-traumatic stress disorder compared to the general population (Gosein, Stifler, Frascoia, & Ford, 2016). Community psychiatrists can serve their formerly incarcerated patients by being sensitive to the potential impact of such an experience and recognizing that work may be needed to establish a strong and supportive therapeutic alliance.

## DISCUSSION

### Background

In the United States, more than 2.2 million individuals, or approximately 1% of the adult population, are incarcerated in jails and prisons (Kaeble, Glaze, Tsoutis, & Minton, 2015). The growth of the incarcerated population is most likely a result, in part, of the confluence of two major initiatives that began in the 1960s: the "war on drugs" and deinstitutionalization from state hospitals. Both of these policy directives significantly affected individuals with mental illness such that now, larger correctional settings such as urban jails and high-capacity prisons have in custody more individuals with mental illness than are admitted to the local state hospitals (Torrey et al., 2014). Males, Black and Hispanic individuals, and those of lower socioeconomic status are overrepresented. Rates of serious mental illness, typically defined as psychotic-spectrum and major mood disorders, along with other diagnoses that cause substantial functional impairment, are estimated to be approximately 14.5% for men and 31% for women in jail (Steadman, Osher, Robbins, Case, & Samuels, 2009). Prisons, which are longer stay institutions designed for individuals convicted of felonies and sentenced to 1 year or more, have a lower prevalence of serious mental illness compared to short-stay jails (James & Glaze, 2006), but they still have rates higher than in the community (Ford, 2015).

### Psychiatric Treatment in a Correctional Setting

Incarcerated individuals are constitutionally entitled to adequate medical and mental health care that originates with the Eighth Amendment of the US Constitution prohibiting cruel and unusual punishment of prisoners (*Estelle v. Gamble*, 1976; *Bowring v. Godwin*, 1977). However, jails and prisons in the United States are not generally considered to be therapeutic environments. Strict rules, limited autonomy, little privacy, and physical and metaphorical isolation from the community are all designed to ensure security but are counterintuitive to what many mental health professionals consider basic requirements for quality care. The abrupt removal from the community to jail with little or no continuity of care, as in the case of Mr. Hernandez, can lead to missed medications, exacerbation of symptoms, delay in diagnosis, and the serious health consequences associated with substance use withdrawal. Mental health staff, who may work for the custodial agency or be independent providers, can struggle with maintaining medical ethical principles in the face of extreme pressure to perform a clinical task for a security goal (e.g., asked to "clear" an individual to go into solitary confinement). At the same time, there can be considerable personal rewards related to the delivery of humane care.

Most correctional settings conduct some form of a mental health and/or suicide risk assessment screen upon admission, with subsequent stratification of services into the equivalent of outpatient care in a clinic setting or residential treatment in specialty mental health housing units. There is typically access to psychiatric infirmaries or inpatient hospital units for those with serious mental illness in acute crisis. Pharmacy formularies may restrict medications because of security concerns; however, there is typically a mechanism to obtain most forms of treatment if clinically necessary. Correctional settings employ a wide range of mental health providers and have variable on-site access to psychiatrists.

Given the prevalence of mental health issues in jails and prisons, increased attention and public health funding have been directed toward improving mental health treatment in these settings. The APA's (2016) third edition of *Psychiatric Services in Correctional Facilities* notes that the "fundamental policy goal for correctional mental health care is to provide the same quality of mental health services to each patient in the criminal justice system as should be available in the community" (p. 5). Accrediting bodies such as the NCCHC are designed to help maintain that quality; however, there is no requirement that correctional settings become accredited. Jails and prisons are funded by local (jails) and state or federal (prisons) governments and are operated either directly through governmental agencies or contracted private vendors. Health care in these settings is typically provided by either independently contracted health care organizations (public or private) or as a component of the relevant DOC agency. Funding for this care also comes from governmental sources (e.g., tax dollars); health insurance (including Medicaid) does not apply in prisons and may only cover the initial 30 days of a jail stay, depending on jurisdiction.

## Continuity of Care upon Release

The vast majority of those who are incarcerated will eventually return to the community in which they were arrested. A critical component of correctional mental health care is planning for an individual's release and establishing treatment connections in the community. However, individuals returning from incarceration may be inappropriately stigmatized as more violent and less clinically appropriate for "regular" and frequently underresourced outpatient clinics that already have long waiting lists. Despite efforts to reduce the practice, it remains common for community treatment providers to refuse enrollment to individuals returning from jail or prison.

While we continue to tackle the triple stigmatization of incarceration, mental illness, and substance use that follow patients who have been in jail or prison, there are practices that can improve the chance of community support. Enrollment in Medicaid while incarcerated, establishing and maintaining a list of quality community providers known to accept individuals returning from jail or prison, and access to statewide Medicaid claims data such as the PSYCKES database in New York can help increase the chance of community engagement.

Correctional psychiatry has been considered a subspecialty of forensic psychiatry, the study of psychiatry and the law; however, it belongs as much, if not more, in the larger field of public psychiatry. Although the ability to deliver patient-centered and effective care in the challenging jail or prison environment requires strong clinical skills and specialized expertise, the patients treated in this system are very much members of local communities. Increased educational opportunities, the expansion of our evidence-based knowledge, and improved provider–provider communication will help minimize the impact of incarceration on individuals with mental health disorders who are overrepresented in these systems.

## REFERENCES

45 Code of Federal Regulations (CFR) Subtitle A,164.152, section k(5).

American Psychiatric Association. (2013). *Diagnostic and statistical manual of mental disorders* (5th ed.). Arlington, VA: American Psychiatric Publishing.

American Psychiatric Association Workgroup to Revise the APA Guidelines on Psychiatric Services in Correctional Facilities. (2016). *Psychiatric services in correctional facilities* (3rd ed.). Arlington, VA: American Psychiatric Publishing.

Baillargeon, J., Binswanger, I. Z., Penn, J. V., Williams, B. A., & Murray, O. J. (2009). Psychiatric disorders and repeat incarcerations: The revolving prison door. *American Journal of Psychiatry, 166*(1), 103–109.

Bowring v. Godwin, 551 F.2d 44, 1977.

Carr, W. A., Rotter, M., Steinbacher, M., Green, T., Dole, T., Garcia-Mansilla, A., . . . Rosenfeld, B. (2006). Structured Assessment of Correctional Adaptation (SACA): A measure of the impact of incarceration on the mentally ill in a therapeutic setting. *International Journal of Offender Therapy and Comparative Criminology, 50*(5), 570–581.

Council of State Governments. (2012). Improving Outcomes for People with Mental Illnesses Involved with New York City's Criminal Court and Correction Systems. http://www.nyc.gov/html/doc/downloads/pdf/press/FINAL_NYC_Report_12_22_2012.pdf

Estelle v. Gamble, 429 U.S. 97, 1976.

Fisher, W. H., Grudzinskas, A. J., Roy-Bujnowski, K. M., & Wolff, N. (2011). Public policy and limits of diversion programs for reducing jail exposure of persons with serious mental illness. *Psychiatric Services, 62*(12), 1503–1505.

Flynn, S., Rodway, C., Appleby, L., & Shaw, J. (2014). Serious violence by people with mental illness: National clinical survey. *Journal of Interpersonal Violence, 29*(8), 1438–1458.

Ford, E. (2015). First-episode psychosis in the criminal justice system: Identifying a critical intercept for early intervention. *Harvard Review of Psychiatry, 23*(3), 167–175.

Gosein, V., Stiffler, J. D., Frascoia, A., & Ford, E. (2016). Life stressors and posttraumatic stress disorder in a seriously mentally ill jail population. *Journal of Forensic Sciences, 61*(1), 116–121.

James, D. J., & Glaze, L. E. (2006). *Mental health problems of prison and jail inmates.* Bureau of Justice Statistics Special Report No. NCJ 213600.

Kaeble, D., Glaze, L., Tsoutis, A., & Minton, T. (2015). *Correctional populations in the United States, 2014.* Bureau of Justice Statistics Special Report No. NCJ249513.

Livingston, J. D. (2016). Contact between police and people with mental disorders: A review of rates. *Psychiatric Services, 67*(8), 850–857.

National Commission on Correctional Health Care. (2014). *Standards for health services in jails.* Chicago, IL: Author.

Noonan, M., Rohloff, H., & Ginder, S. (2015). *Mortality in local jails and state prisons, 2000–2013—Statistical tables.* Bureau of Justice Statistics Special Report No. NCJ248756.

Nunn, A., Zaller, N., Dickman, S., Trimbur, C., Nijhawan, A., & Rich, J. D. (2009). Methadone and buprenorphine prescribing and referral practices in U.S. prison systems: Results from a nationwide survey. *Drug and Alcohol Dependence*, *105*(1–2), 83–88.

Steadman, H. J., Osher, F. C., Robbins, P. C., Case, B., & Samuels, S. (2009). Prevalence of serious mental illness among jail inmates. *Psychiatric Services*, *60*, 761–765.

Torrey, E. F., Zdanowicz, M. T., Kennard, A. D., Lamb, H. R., Eslinger, D. F., & Biasotti, M. C. (2014). *The treatment of persons with mental illness in prisons and jails: A state survey*. Treatment Advocacy Center. Retrieved from http://www.treatmentadvocacycenter.org/the-treatment-of-persons-with-mental-illness-in-prisons-and-jails-2014/state-results. Accessed June 15, 2016.

# 19

# Homelessness

### JOANNA FRIED AND LEORA MORINIS ∎

## CASE HISTORY

Anthony is a 49-year-old multiracial man who has been street homeless for the past 8 years. He recently began engaging with a street outreach team on which you work as a psychiatric provider. He is scheduled to see you for an evaluation for the purposes of applying for supportive housing. His outreach case manager reminds him about his 10 a.m. appointment with you. He arrives at the office at 3:30 p.m., and when told you are meeting with another consumer, he storms out of the office. The next morning, you and his outreach case manager visit him in the field, and you introduce yourself. He says he is on his way to a food pantry but accepts your card. He agrees to return to your office, and his outreach case manager gives him bus fare so he will be able to travel.

### Clinical Pearl

Many people confronting homelessness are juggling competing demands for their time, attention, and resources. Their priorities may be different than those of the people working with them. This can be challenging to practitioners trained to work within a well-defined treatment frame. It can take several attempts before someone will meet with a psychiatrist, and engagement may involve meeting with people on a park bench, at a shelter, or at a food pantry or providing transportation to an office. Even once a treatment relationship is established, appointment times need to be flexible, no-shows or "drop-in" visits should be expected, and a clinician's services may include care coordination, advocacy, outreach, and crisis intervention. Programs serving individuals experiencing homelessness need to build flexibility into practitioners' schedules. To allow for effective interventions, caseloads may need to be lower, and traditional measures of "productivity" may not be suitable.

Anthony shows up that afternoon. He explains that he initially became homeless when he was 16 years old; he had a conflictual relationship with his stepfather, who was physically abusive to his mother. He went to stay with an older girlfriend in a rented room. He left school and joined a neighborhood gang. He was arrested for the first time when he was 17 for selling marijuana and served a 3-year prison term. When he was released, his family would not allow him to stay with them, so he entered the shelter system. During the next 25 years, Anthony was in and out of incarceration (often for parole violations or minor infractions related to homelessness), the shelter system, emergency rooms, psychiatric inpatient units, and substance abuse treatment programs. His current 8-year period of street homelessness began when he was discharged from a long-term residential substance abuse treatment program after a physical altercation with another consumer. He says he did not re-enter the shelter system because he did not feel safe in shelters: "They're crowded and dirty and people in there are smoking crack and stealing from each other."

Anthony explains that he had a "couple of drinks" on his way to meet with you. He says he drinks "a few beers" daily with friends in the park. This represents a decrease from last year, when he was drinking a pint of vodka daily. He has been smoking cannabis daily since age 13 and recently started smoking synthetic cannabinoids (known as "K2" or "spice") because it is less expensive and easily accessible.

When asked about psychiatric history, Anthony says "I've always been moody" and that he has a "hot temper" and limited patience. As a child, he was often in trouble at school and at home because, he explains, "I got bored easily and liked to keep moving." He endorses periodic episodes, since his twenties, of feeling "stressed" and experiencing low mood and motivation, insomnia, feelings of hopelessness and worthlessness, and passive suicidal ideation (although he says, "I would never do that to myself"). When asked about mania, he says his mind is often racing and that he never sleeps more than 2 or 3 hours at a time, but he denies feeling tired. During your meeting, he is friendly and well-related, his speech is rapid (although not pressured), and he often gets out of his seat to emphasize a point. He is at times circumstantial, going into great detail when telling stories about his past, but he is easily redirected.

### Clinical Pearl

It can be challenging to evaluate and diagnose individuals in homeless services settings; practitioners often have limited time to do a full evaluation and little access to collateral information, medical workup, or diagnostic testing. In these circumstances, it can be difficult to narrow a differential diagnosis or to determine how much substance use may contribute to current or past psychiatric symptoms. When possible (and with the client's consent), accessing statewide Medicaid databases, asking support staff to obtain prior treatment records, and seeking collateral information from community members and service providers can help refine the diagnostic process.

Anthony explains that he saw a psychiatrist for the first time when he was 9 years old and having behavioral issues at school and subsequently when incarcerated or in substance abuse treatment programs. He says he has been diagnosed "bipolar schizophrenic" and "antisocial" and has been hospitalized "a few times." He has been prescribed psychiatric medications on multiple occasions but cannot remember details, although he recalls that he was treated with Thorazine during one hospitalization. While taking it, he felt like a "zombie" and could not focus his thoughts, but he says "a judge forced me to take it." He explains that when he had refused, the inpatient team went to court for treatment over objection.

## Clinical Pearl

Psychopharmacology with individuals who are homeless requires a mix of flexibility, creativity, and patience. People who are living on the street often do not have a safe place to keep medications and may be wary about side effects that might impair their ability to stay alert. Benefits, including health insurance, are often unstable or inactive, making it difficult to start or maintain a medication regimen. They have reduced access to primary care or laboratory services, so it may be challenging to fill or refill prescriptions, monitor blood levels or metabolic impact, or address medication side effects. The use of lower doses of medications, pharmaceutical company patient-assistance programs, and long-acting injectable antipsychotics can all help improve adherence and access to medication.

Anthony agrees to meet with you once a week while the outreach team works on his housing; he says, "I don't mind talking to you but I'm not going to take any pills." As you get to know him, you learn that although he went to school through the 10th grade, he is largely unable to read. Nonetheless, he managed to get his Commercial Driver's License and drove a tractor trailer for a year in his twenties. At another point, he taught himself basic electrical repair and now sometimes restores electronic equipment he finds in the trash. During one visit, he comments that your office is dim, and the next week he brings you a desk lamp he repaired. He describes himself as "very protective" of others, often recounting the ways he provides support to other street homeless individuals in his community.

## Clinical Pearl

It is often simple to identify the many deficits of individuals experiencing homelessness, mental illness, and substance abuse. However, these same individuals often have extraordinary resources and resilience. Despite trauma, loss, and challenging circumstances, they manage to survive, develop coping strategies, and navigate complex systems. It can be helpful from early on to identify an individual's talents and adaptive coping mechanisms and to work using a strengths-based model.

After several weeks of meeting with him, he appears withdrawn and dysphoric and reports that he is having an episode of "the blues." He says it is becoming difficult to motivate himself to stick to his daily routine. He has no appetite, and he feels like he will be homeless "forever." This continues for 2 weeks, and he misses his next appointment with you. The team locates him and brings him to the office one afternoon—he is intoxicated, tearful, and says he is being followed by members of the gang he left when he was 19 years old. He says they are leaving him "signs," explaining that several dents appeared on the mailbox on the corner where he sleeps. He reveals he has been thinking about jumping off a bridge and describes a plan to do so. You confer with the outreach team and decide he is at high risk for self-harm and requires evaluation at an emergency room. You discuss this with Anthony, who refuses, saying "If you call the cops on me, I'll disappear." You explain that you and the team are concerned for his safety and that if he is willing to go to the emergency room, his outreach case manager will accompany him and you will speak to the doctor on call. He agrees, but he is only willing to go to the hospital where he was treated for cellulitis because, he says, the staff treated him with respect.

### Clinical Pearl

An overwhelming percentage of individuals experiencing homelessness have a history of exposure to trauma. Moreover, homelessness itself is traumatic and often represents the end product of multiple losses—the loss of not only a home but also community, identity, stability, and physical safety. Anthony has not told you details about his time in the gang but has alluded to witnessing significant violence—at home, on the streets, and while incarcerated. Even in individuals who do not meet diagnostic criteria for post-traumatic stress disorder, trauma exposure can impact psychosocial functioning in a number of ways and can compound diagnostic complexity. Anthony's history of trauma exposure may contribute to affective instability, paranoid ideation, difficulty with relationships, substance use, and other ongoing difficulties. Understanding these challenges and exploring the impact of trauma when working with people who are homeless can help inform diagnosis and treatment.

Anthony is admitted to the inpatient psychiatric unit. You and his case manager visit him. On medication, his mood improves and his psychotic symptoms abate. You advocate for a long-acting injectable antipsychotic, which Anthony agrees to. Upon discharge, the outreach team secures him a private room in a local "safe haven" that has an onsite psychiatrist. He sees you once more in the office; you then visit the safe haven, where you and he meet the psychiatrist there to discuss his treatment and future. Three months later, he stops by the office to show you the keys to his apartment; he has moved into supportive housing. He reports that it has been a challenging transition and that he is grateful that the outreach team has continued to meet with him weekly for the past 3 months. He is participating in a nearby rehabilitation program. He tells you he stopped taking the injectable antipsychotic because it made his arm sore, but he is now taking oral medication. His building offers medication administration support, and staff help him pack a weekly pillbox.

## DISCUSSION

### Background

According to the US Department of Housing and Urban Development (HUD, 2016), on one night in January 2016, 549,928 people in the United States were homeless; more than one-fifth (22%) of these were children younger than age 18. A small but significant minority (14%) meet HUD criteria for chronic homelessness: being homeless for 1 year or more or having 4 or more episodes of homelessness in the past

3 years, and also having a disabling condition (HUD, 2016). The chronically homeless often have higher rates of behavioral health problems and are frequent users of expensive services such as emergency rooms, crisis response, and incarceration. Homelessness and incarceration are mutual risk factors for each other (Greenberg & Rosenheck, 2008). Substance abuse and severe mental illness—both more prevalent among people experiencing homelessness than in the general population—are associated with increased risk of criminal justice involvement.

It has been consistently estimated that between one-third and one-half of people experiencing homelessness have mental illness (McQuistion, 2012), and a recent meta-analysis of studies between 1966 and 2007 from Western countries found prevalence of 37.9% for alcohol dependence and 24.4% for other substance dependence (Fazel, Khosla, Doll, & Geddes, 2008). In addition, homeless individuals are often at a disproportionately high risk for infectious disease and trauma-related injuries, along with metabolic and respiratory disorders (Badiaga, Raoult, & Brouqui, 2008).

## Evidence-Based and Innovative Practices

### HOUSING FIRST
This approach provides permanent, independent housing for chronically homeless individuals who have serious mental illness and/or substance use disorders, without prerequisites for sobriety or participation in treatment. Compared to more traditional methods of housing (sometimes called "treatment first"), which rely on a linear step-by-step continuum to "housing readiness," Housing First has a higher retention rate, reduces the use of costly emergency and crisis services, and creates a more stable foundation from which individuals can begin to address other issues (Aubry, Nelson, & Tsemberis, 2015)

### PERMANENT SUPPORTIVE HOUSING
Permanent supportive housing is safe, affordable housing that is integrated into the community and offers flexible support. Tenants in this type of housing typically have access to ongoing case management designed to support them in maintaining housing and addressing current needs. In some supportive housing, onsite services may include psychiatric and medical care, medication administration support, and/or meals. There is evidence for the success of permanent supportive housing for individuals with homelessness, psychiatric illness, and substance use disorders. Compared to other models of treatment, it reduces homelessness, increases housing stability, and decreases emergency room use and hospitalization. Consumers consistently rate permanent supportive housing more positively than other housing models (Rog et al., 2014).

### INTEGRATED TREATMENT FOR CO-OCCURRING DISORDERS
There is substantial literature supporting the use of integrated treatment for individuals who are homeless and have co-occurring psychiatric and substance abuse disorders. Providing coordinated services can improve multiple outcomes, including psychiatric hospitalizations, substance abuse, and housing (Substance Abuse and Mental Health Services Administration, 2013). Psychopharmacological treatment

of substance use disorders with medications such as naltrexone and buprenorphine can help reduce harm and support recovery.

### CRITICAL TIME INTERVENTION

Critical Time Intervention (CTI) is time-limited, targeted, and intensive case management designed to prevent homelessness for individuals in vulnerable transition situations (e.g., transition from shelter to permanent housing, discharge from long-term psychiatric hospitalization, or release from incarceration). Case managers provide support before, during, and after the transition in order to keep the client engaged and to prevent homelessness or worsening of behavioral health problems. Randomized trials have demonstrated that CTI has a meaningful and lasting ability to reduce the risk of homelessness for people with serious mental illness returning to the community (Herman et al., 2011).

### TRAUMA-INFORMED CARE

Being homeless increases the risk of further traumatization (Hopper, Bassuk, & Oliver, 2010). The impact of traumatic stress can be devastating and can interfere with an individual's sense of safety, perception of control, ability to self-regulate, and ability to form healthy interpersonal relationships. When working with people experiencing homelessness, it is important to ask about a history of trauma and consider how it may impact current functioning. Providing trauma-informed services to patients who are homeless includes using shared decision-making to return some sense of control over their circumstances (for further information, see Chapter 2).

## Systems Challenges

The funding for homeless services varies by location but often relies on a combination of government and private resources, which makes it vulnerable to changes in public opinion as well as trends in policy and politics. The limited availability of affordable housing poses a great challenge in treating homeless individuals. Permanent and temporary supportive housing facilities are often in short supply, and states must often find creative solutions to fund and expand supportive housing. One solution is the use of Medicaid to develop supportive housing and fund associated case management services, as has been done in New York State.

Limited treatment availability also presents a significant challenge. There is a shortage of mental health treatment options in general, and there are significant barriers to access for homeless individuals. These barriers include not having a fixed address, not being able to keep defined appointment times, and lacking money for or access to transportation.

The case discussed in this chapter illustrates the importance of specialized approaches for clinical work with homeless individuals. Many individuals without housing are not well served within the existing outpatient mental health services system. Without tailored interventions, many cannot or do not access ongoing psychiatric care. Team-based and integrated approaches that include street and shelter outreach and address housing, mental and physical health, substance use, and benefits and entitlements are most likely to be successful.

# REFERENCES

Aubry, T., Nelson, G., & Tsemberis, S. (2015). Housing First for people with severe mental illness who are homeless: A review of the research and findings from the At Home–Chez soi demonstration project. *Canadian Journal of Psychiatry, 60*(11), 467–474.

Badiaga, S., Raoult, D., & Brouqui, P. (2008). Preventing and controlling emerging and reemerging transmissible diseases in the homeless. *Emerging Infectious Diseases, 14*(9), 1353–1359.

Fazel, S., Khosla, V., Doll, H., & Geddes, J. (2008). The prevalence of mental disorders among the homeless in Western countries: Systematic review and meta-regression analysis. *PLoS Medicine, 5*(12), 1670–1681. doi:10.1371/journal.pmed.0050225

Greenberg, G. A., & Rosenheck, R. A. (2008). Jail incarceration, homelessness, and mental health: A national study. *Psychiatric Services, 59*(2), 170–177. doi:10.1176/ps.2008.59.2.170

Herman, D. B., Conover, S., Gorroochurn, P., Hinterland, K., Hoepner, L., & Susser, E. S. (2011). Randomized trial of critical time intervention to prevent homelessness after hospital discharge. *Psychiatric Services, 62*(7), 713–719. doi:10.1176/appi.ps.62.7.713

Hopper, E. K., Bassuk, E. L., & Oliver, J. (2010). Shelter from the storm: Trauma-informed care in homeless services settings. *The Open Health Services and Policy Journal, 3*, 80–100.

McQuistion, H. L. (2012). Homeless and behavioral health in the new century. In H. L. McQuistion, W. E. Sowers, J. M. Ranz, & J. M. Feldman (Eds.), *Handbook of community psychiatry* (pp. 407–422). New York, NY: Springer.

Rog, D. J., Marshall, T., Dougherty, R. H., George, P., Daniels, A. S., Ghose, S. S., & Delphin-Rittmon, M. E. (2014). Permanent supportive housing: Assessing the evidence. *Psychiatric Services, 65*(3), 287–294. doi:10.1176/appi.ps.201300261

Substance Abuse and Mental Health Services Administration. (2013). *Behavioral health services for people who are homeless.* Treatment Improvement Protocol (TIP) Series No. 55. (HHS Publication No. (SMA) 13-4734. Rockville, MD: Author.

US Department of Housing and Urban Development. (2016). *2016 annual homeless assessment report (2016 AHAR) to Congress.* Washington, DC: Author.

# 20

# Co-occurring Substance Use Disorders

## MICHAEL SOULE AND HILARY S. CONNERY ∎

### CASE HISTORY

Mr. Jones is a 49-year-old man who presents as a referral from his new primary care physician (PCP) with complaints of depressed mood. Because he recently lost his job and health insurance, he lost his previous provider and has come to your city hospital for care. His medical history is significant for mild hypertension and obesity. Your hospital recently instituted an initiative to screen primary care patients with the Patient Health Questionnaire-9. He scored 16 of 27 points possible, endorsing depressed mood, difficulty sleeping, loss of motivation, and some thoughts that he would be better off dead but with no active suicidal planning. An 8-week trial with a selective serotonin reuptake inhibitor (SSRI) did not improve his reported symptoms; in fact, he appeared to be progressively more impaired, prompting a referral to the behavioral health clinic.

As part of your comprehensive history, you learn that Mr. Jones first suffered from what he describes as "light" depression as a teen. During a stressful period in high school, he saw a counselor, which he found helpful. After he married at age 25, he would have occasional episodes of melancholy but nothing significant or long-lasting. Two years ago, his wife left him for another man. Since then, he has experienced progressively depressed mood, loneliness, and neurovegetative symptoms consistent with a major depressive episode.

Single-item screening for alcohol and drug use in the past year is positive for alcohol only, and when you administer the brief version of the Alcohol Use Disorders Identification Test (AUDIT-C), he scores 10 of 12 possible points. He further discloses that at night he drinks wine to help him sleep, typically consuming one or two 750-mL bottles nightly.

### Clinical Pearl

AUDIT-C is a brief screening tool to identify problem drinking (Bush, et al., 1998) with the following questions:

- How often do you have a drink containing alcohol?
- How many standard drinks containing alcohol do you have on a typical day?
- How often do you have six or more drinks on one occasion?

A standard drink is defined as containing 10 grams of ethanol, such that 12 ounces of beer is equivalent to 5 ounces of wine or 1.5 ounces of liquor. An AUDIT-C screening score greater than or equal to 4 for men and 3 for women is considered positive for hazardous drinking. Further review of diagnostic criteria for alcohol use disorder is warranted in such cases.

Mr. Jones states that in the past month, there were 4 days when he did not drink, with the longest consecutive alcohol-free period lasting 2 days. He has never had symptoms of withdrawal and has no prior treatment history. He denies driving while intoxicated.

## Clinical Pearl

A thorough safety evaluation includes assessment of symptoms of alcohol withdrawal during abstinent periods, suggesting need for medically monitored detoxification, as well as assessment of machinery or motor vehicle operation while under the influence and caring for minors or dependents while intoxicated. Even if patients are drinking heavily, if they have not exhibited symptoms of alcohol withdrawal during abstinence and they are younger than age 70 years, it is generally safe to treat them in a monitored outpatient setting. Some medical comorbidities that would preclude outpatient-based treatment include autonomic instability, uncontrolled hypertension, and diabetes mellitus.

In further conversation, you learn that Mr. Jones believes his drinking patterns are unhealthy, but because he never has needed a drink in the morning and has been able to abstain from drinking for a night or two, he believes he can "quit whenever he wants." However, he wonders if he will sleep and how he will cope with loneliness if he gives up drinking.

## Clinical Pearl

Motivational interviewing (MI) is a patient-centered approach to behavioral change. Instead of assuming that Mr. Jones' drinking is a problem and diving right into a discussion of his habits, the clinician using an MI style will ask him for permission to have a conversation about his drinking. This allows respect for the patient's autonomy, capacity, and responsibility for considering health-related behavioral changes. MI serves the purpose of clarifying the patient's personal goals and values and assisting the patient in the process of making changes to support these goals and values. A fundamental MI skill is the use of "reflective listening," a manner of reflecting back to the patient what you hear him or her communicating. For Mr. Jones, you might reflect at this point, "Your drinking is somewhat of a problem, but you really enjoy drinking and aren't sure you want to cut down." This serves both to clarify that you have understood the patient accurately and to move the dialogue in the direction of an open, honest, and confidential discussion related to options for change.

Mr. Jones discloses that he first drank alcohol at age 19 and never was a daily drinker until his divorce. He began to "treat" himself to a couple of glasses of wine at night to "drown [his] sorrows." Eventually, he would just finish the bottle. He shares that at this point, he noticed that his drinking had become a nightly pattern. You reflect back, "When you started to finish the bottle of wine, you really noticed your drinking had increased." He nods and says, "I worried I was becoming an alcoholic, but I was too down to care."

At his request, you provide psychoeducation about depression and alcohol use, and Mr. Jones remarks that he noticed his mood getting worse during that period but believed it was related to the divorce. You offer that reducing or stopping drinking will likely help both his mood and his blood pressure, and you ask if he would like to learn about medications that can help with reducing drinking. He agrees.

### Clinical Pearl

Medication-assisted treatment (MAT) pairs medication for a substance use disorder with psychoeducation and a structured, goal-directed behavioral treatment plan to reduce substance use. In the United States, three US Food and Drug Administration (FDA)-approved medications to treat alcohol use disorder are naltrexone, acamprosate, and disulfiram. Naltrexone, a mu-opioid antagonist, reduces the reinforcing central effect of alcohol consumption, such that a person intending to abstain from drinking will experience less reward with taking a drink, thereby helping prevent a "slip" from turning into a full relapse episode. A long-acting depot formulation of naltrexone is available for patients for whom adherence may be a concern. Acamprosate appears to work by normalizing alcohol-related changes in gamma-aminobutyric acid and glutamate signaling, which supports patient self-regulation during early abstinence. Disulfiram, an aldehyde dehydrogenase inhibitor, interferes with alcohol metabolism and causes acetaldehyde toxicity if the person consumes alcohol. Studies show that enlisting a patient's family in witnessed administration of disulfiram improves medication adherence and family relations. Topiramate is not currently FDA approved, but it has a robust evidence base for improving drinking outcomes, and it acts as a partial substitute for alcohol-related changes in neural signaling.

MAT is also available for opioid use disorders (i.e., buprenorphine, methadone, and extended-release naltrexone) and nicotine use disorders (nicotine replacement, bupropion, and varenicline). MAT is discussed in greater detail in Chapter 5. Unfortunately, little evidence supports MAT for other substance use disorders at this time.

You discuss a behavioral plan. Mr. Jones will aim to reduce from five to eight glasses of wine nightly to four or five glasses per night. He agrees to track his drinking volume and frequency daily. You draw a hepatic panel to determine if adjunctive naltrexone will be safely tolerated, further increase his SSRI dose to treat depression, and prescribe a non-benzodiazepine medication to assist with sleep onset as needed. You would also recommend cognitive–behavioral therapy (CBT) to support recovery, but you are unable to locate an available therapist who also accepts public health insurance. You discuss mutual help organizations, including Alcoholics Anonymous (AA) and Smart Recovery. Mr. Jones commits to trying AA, and you examine the website together for meetings in his area. You offer him a menu of smartphone apps with which to monitor cravings, mood, and sleep. You discuss referral to your clinic's recovery coach program, in which people with a lived experience of recovery have been clinically trained to support patient efforts to achieve sobriety.

After Mr. Jones signs a release of information, you speak with Mr. Jones' PCP, letting her know your findings about his alcohol consumption. She expresses some surprise and then says, "Well I guess we know why he's depressed! We can stop the antidepressant until he's been sober for a while and then we can really see what's going on with his depression."

### Clinical Pearl

When a mood disorder and substance use disorder are co-occurring, it is often not possible to predict the impact of substance abstinence on the symptoms of the co-occurring mood disorder. Sometimes a prior history of symptom continuation during a period of abstinence will confirm the diagnosis of a mood disorder, but often the history and presentation are less clear. When a mood disorder is accompanied by significant thoughts of suicide or other self-harm behaviors, it is considered dangerous to withhold medical care for the mood disorder. In controlled, highly monitored settings such as residential or partial hospital programs, it may be safe and rational to assess the impact of abstinence on the mood symptoms; however, when treating dual-diagnosis patients in outpatient community settings, this approach may be ineffective if there are limits to a patient's access to re-evaluation and medical intervention. If you suspect that a mood disorder is substance-induced but follow-up is not timely, prescribing medication to address both substance and mood disorders is recommended with the option of later reducing the psychotropic medication if substance abstinence results in sustained recovery.

When Mr. Jones returns for follow-up, he indicates that his mood is slightly better, but cutting down on drinking has been more challenging than he anticipated. You inform him that his liver transaminases are within normal limits and that naltrexone would be an option. He relates that he has difficulty adhering to daily medication regimens and likes the idea of a once-monthly depot naltrexone injection. Your clinic does not administer the medication due to the administrative burden. There is another clinic in the area that does provide injections, but it would require him to receive all his care there; he prefers to remain in current care and use a pillbox and reminders to support medication adherence.

## DISCUSSION

### Prevalence

Among people with any mental illness, nearly one in five have a co-occurring substance use disorder, and treatment-seeking community prevalence rates are higher (30–55%), particularly within more intensive levels of care (Center for Behavioral Health Statistics and Quality [CBHSQ], 2015; Grant et al., 2004; Rush & Koegl, 2008). Severity of mental illness is associated positively with frequency of alcohol and drug use disorders (CBHSQ, 2015). Childhood adversity is significantly associated with future onset of mental health and substance use disorder and is considered an important target for primary prevention (McLaughlin et al., 2012). The case in this chapter details the common scenario of co-occurring depression and alcohol use disorder; co-occurring serious mental illnesses including schizophrenia or bipolar disorder present additional complexities, as do the use of illicit drugs including opioids, which have reached epidemic proportions, and the use of newer drugs (e.g., synthetic cannabinoids) with less predictable effects.

### Models of Care

Collaborative care is the community standard for the treatment of co-occurring disorders, using either a parallel system of coordination (e.g., collaboration between community mental health center staff working with opioid treatment program staff for a patient receiving mental health and methadone maintenance therapies) or, ideally, fully integrated treatment within one system (e.g., the availability of office-based treatment with buprenorphine/naloxone allows integrated treatment of co-occurring opioid use disorder within a community mental health center). The traditional model of achieving abstinence from substance use prior to initiating treatment of a co-occurring mental illness is not supported by empirical evidence and is also not practical, given the high dropout rates with this approach.

### Treatment Engagement and Retention

All mental health disorders, including substance use disorders, are chronic illnesses that have in common a pathology of thought process (ranging from distortion to frank thought disorder) and a pathology of stress reactivity (which may be hypo- or hyperfunctional). This syndrome results in challenges within social and occupational functioning and disturbances of behavioral self-regulation. Impairments related to mental health disorders are highly stigmatized and frequently misperceived as volitional impairments rather than as neurobiological deficits. The most vital aspect for patient care is the successful engagement of patients in treatment and the successful retention of patients in longitudinal maintenance therapies. This is of increased importance with increased comorbidity because dropout rates are higher and outcomes are poorer for those with increased burden of illness (Brunette & Mueser, 2006). Successful engagement and retention results from creating a highly confidential and patient-centered environment within which clinicians are able to skillfully apply evidence-based practices such as MI, contingency management, CBT, mindfulness-based therapies, supported employment, peer support, case management, and rapid access to medication-assisted treatments. Removing barriers to transportation and child care and having mobile and residence-based services available to reach disadvantaged populations (e.g., homeless and elderly) will enhance treatment outcomes and quality of care delivered.

## System Challenges

Three major challenges continue to detract from optimal care of those with co-occurring disorders. The first challenge is fragmentation: Divisions between payment streams for "physical health," "mental health," and "substance abuse" treatments produce false barriers between service lines that must be overcome in order to care optimally for this population with complex needs. Co-location and coordination of services can help remedy these splits. Related to this, payment systems' limits on services (e.g., visit frequency or access to case management) and medical formulary may demand that a given patient's condition worsen before he or she is able to access an indicated service intensity. Once this threshold is met, patients then often face wait lists. Larger organizations may be able to circumvent these limitations by cross-subsidizing needed services according to clinician assessment rather than payer determinations.

Second, most clinical trials for medications targeting mental health/substance use disorders exclude patients with co-occurring disorders. Relative to the literature on each set of disorders in isolation, the literature on co-occurring disorders is thin (Pettinati, O'Brien, & Dundon, 2013). The paucity of studies in the field precludes replication of findings and establishment of firm guidelines. It may be difficult to distinguish whether a primary mood disorder is contributing to a substance use disorder; whether the opposite is true; or whether they are related cyclically, with each entity worsening the other (Pettinati et al., 2013).

A third challenge has been the implementation of evidence-based psychosocial treatments for mental health/substance use disorders. Both contingency management and CBT are strongly evidence-based but have been underutilized given their demonstrated efficacy. Contingency management programs incent healthy behaviors with cash, gift cards, privileges, or other incentives. Due to federal and state prohibitions for incentivizing service utilization, only a handful of states have launched creative incentive-based programs through Medicaid, aimed broadly at incentivizing various health behaviors (Hand, Heil, Sigmon, & Higgins, 2014). Implementation of CBT is limited in large part by the unavailability of reimbursed training and longitudinal supervision required for treatment fidelity (Carroll, 2014). In addition, wide variability in access to and quality of community-based CBT remains problematic. MI, by contrast, tends to be more readily disseminated and implemented by professional and paraprofessional staff in community settings, facilitating treatment and supporting the change efforts of those with co-occurring disorders.

REFERENCES

Brunette, M. F., & Mueser, K. T. (2006). Psychosocial interventions for the long-term management of patients with severe mental illness and co-occurring substance use disorder. *Journal of Clinical Psychiatry*, *67*(Suppl. 7), 10–17.

Bush, K., Kivlahan, D. R., McDonell, M. B., Fihn, S. D., & Bradley, K. A. (1998). The AUDIT alcohol consumption questions (AUDIT-C): An effective brief screening test for problem drinking. *Archives of Internal Medicine*, *158*(16), 1789–1795.

Carroll, K. M. (2014). Lost in translation? Moving contingency management and cognitive behavioral therapy into clinical practice. *Annals of the New York Academy of Sciences*, *1327*, 94–111.

Center for Behavioral Health Statistics and Quality. (2015). *2014 National survey on drug use and health: Mental health detailed tables*. Rockville, MD: Substance Abuse and Mental Health Services Administration. Retrieved from https://www.samhsa.gov/data/sites/default/files/NSDUH-DetTabs2014/NSDUH-DetTabs2014.pdf. Accessed November 29, 2015.

Grant, B. F., Stinson, F. S., Dawson, D. A., Chou, P., Dufour, M. C., Compton, W., . . . Kaplan, K. (2004). Prevalence and co-occurrence of substance use disorders and independent mood and anxiety disorders: Results from the National Epidemiologic Survey on Alcohol and Related Conditions. *Archives of General Psychiatry*, *61*(8), 807–816.

Hand, D. J., Heil, S. H., Sigmon, S. C., & Higgins, S. T. (2014). Improving Medicaid health incentives programs: Lessons from substance abuse treatment research. *Preventive Medicine*, *63*, 87–89.

McLaughlin, K. A., Greif Green, J., Gruber, M. J., Sampson, N. A., Zaslavsky, A. M., & Kessler, R. C. (2012). Childhood adversities and first onset of psychiatric disorders in a national sample of US adolescents. *Archives of General Psychiatry*, *69*(11), 1151–1160.

Pettinati, H. M., O'Brien, C. P., & Dundon, W. D. (2013). Current status of co-occurring mood and substance use disorders: A new therapeutic target. *American Journal of Psychiatry*, *170*(1), 23–30.

Rush, B., & Koegl, C. J. (2008). Prevalence and profile of people with co-occurring mental and substance use disorders within a comprehensive mental health system. *Canadian Journal of Psychiatry*, *53*(12), 810–821.

# 21

# Individuals with Developmental Disabilities

KATHARINE STRATIGOS, NINA TIOLECO, ANNA SILBERMAN, AND AGNES WHITAKER ∎

## CASE HISTORY

Daniel is an 18-year-old young man who is currently in the psychiatric emergency department (ED). The ED admission diagnoses are unspecified disruptive disorder (serious aggression) and autism spectrum disorder (ASD) with accompanying intellectual impairment and language impairment.

You have come to the ED to learn more about him before he is transferred to the inpatient unit, where you will lead the team caring for him. You are directed to a heavyset young man of average height; he is sitting on a stretcher, hospital gown askew, slouched over a computer tablet. When you introduce yourself, he peers at your ID card and mumbles your name. He seems fixated on his computer tablet, playing and replaying the same section of a muted Disney video. When lunch arrives, he looks up toward you but seems to stare through you. You note that he uses eating utensils appropriately. After he is finished eating, he repeatedly arches his back, flaps both hands at shoulder level, and suddenly rocks forward, smiling slightly. You notice that he is looking intently at the menu choices for dinner, and you wonder if he can read.

### Clinical Pearl

Autism spectrum disorder has two core criteria: (1) persistent, cross-situational deficits in social communication and social interaction and (2) restricted and repetitive behaviors, interests, and activities; symptoms of both are manifest in early life (American Psychiatric Association [APA], 2013). However, there is no "typical" clinical presentation of ASD. Each patient's presentation varies based on the severity of signs, intellectual and language impairments, and associated medical and psychiatric features.

ASD, which currently affects 1.5% of school-age children in the United States (Lyall et al., 2017), is one of the five specific "neurodevelopmental disorders" in

DSM-5. The others are intellectual disabilities (1%), communication disorders (6%), attention deficit hyperactivity disorder (ADHD; 5%), specific learning disorders (5–15%), and motor disorders (e.g., developmental coordination disorder; 5–6%) (APA, 2013). They are grouped together because the signs that define them are apparent very early in life and because they are associated with atypical brain development during that period. Each of these disorders commonly co-occurs with one or more other neurodevelopmental disorders. Intellectual disabilities, communication disorders, and ADHD each occur in approximately one-third of people with ASD (Lyall et al., 2017; Wodka, Mathy, & Kalb, 2013). Language disabilities complicate the ED assessment, especially in nonverbal persons with ASD (e.g., functional use of fewer than five single words). In nonverbal patients, IQ may not reflect their problem-solving abilities because most IQ measures are language based. Alternative methods of communication, including pictures, sign language, and the written word, are possible. Computers can be especially helpful for those whose motor problems make signing or handwriting difficult.

After a chart review and speaking with staff, you learn that Daniel had been living with his elderly grandparents, who are immigrants and do not speak English. They became his legal guardians when he was a toddler, after his single mother physically abused him.

On the evening of the current ED admission, Daniel's grandmother had called 911 after Daniel struck his grandfather, who had been helping him take a shower. Daniel calmed down immediately in the ED. History revealed that he had been brought to the same ED for aggression approximately once a month during the past year. Once in the ED, his aggression would abate quickly without other interventions, and he would be discharged home. However, just prior to this admission, Daniel had turned 18 years old. His grandparents had not applied to be his legal guardians past his 18th birthday. Although they loved him dearly, they felt very unsafe and overwhelmed by his aggressive outbursts. They no longer felt able to be legally responsible for him, especially because they both now had serious health problems.

His grandparents are eager to tell you that Daniel is generally a quiet, gentle person. When he was a child, he had occasional temper tantrums at home, usually occurring when he was asked to transition from one activity to another or when asked to bathe (he has a strong sensory aversion to water). As he entered adolescence, his temper outbursts began to frighten them. In order to prevent outbursts, they largely abandoned efforts to transition him from one activity or another at home and allowed him to shower infrequently. Over time, his outbursts in response to any transition or to showering at all increased in severity and frequency. At 5 feet 10 inches and 225 pounds, his outbursts put others at risk. Recently, when his grandmother attempted to take his computer tablet away before bedtime, he pushed her into a chair; she sustained a serious scalp laceration that required stitches. Striking his grandfather in the shower, to the point of bruising him, brought them to this crisis point. You note that he did not have temper outbursts or aggression at school.

## Clinical Pearl

Aggression is a nonspecific behavior, more common in persons with ASD than in their typically developing or intellectually disabled peers. Effective treatment of aggression in ASD is best accomplished by systematically assessing contributing factors and addressing them in an individualized treatment plan (McGuire et al., 2016). The six sets of factors to be considered are (1) medical conditions, (2) functional communication problems, (3) psychosocial stressors, (4) maladaptive patterns of reinforcement by caretakers, (5) psychiatric disorders, and (6) irritability and aggression associated with ASD.

Always rule out medical conditions causing pain or discomfort. This requires a complete review of systems with both caretakers and the patient and a physical exam. Prompt treatment of a tooth abscess or of fecal impaction, for example, may be the sole intervention required. Now considered standard of care for ASD, consider genetic testing, especially in a patient with dysmorphic features; certain genetic syndromes carry specific behavioral phenotypes that may help clarify behavioral presentation.

Co-occurring psychiatric disorders may be difficult to diagnose in persons with ASD because of cognitive or language impairments. The most common psychiatric disorders to accompany ASD are anxiety disorders, ADHD, and obsessive–compulsive disorder (Murphy et al., 2016).

Once Daniel is on the inpatient unit, your team notes that he does not interact with the other patients at all. He is not asked to participate in groups due to his spoken language impairment, but he becomes irritable and slightly agitated when staff tell him that it is time to transition from one room or activity to another. Thinking it might be helpful, his grandparents bring his computer tablet from home. Inpatient rules, however, do not allow unrestricted access to his computer tablet. He becomes angry when staff gesture that it is time for him to put it away, and he grabs at their arms, saying "no" loudly.

The staff also note that Daniel is spending increasing amounts of time in the bathroom. When staff members do their usual 15-minute check, knocking and verbally inquiring as to how he is, he emerges with his pants down and his hands up. Some staff feel frightened by this behavior. When staff and security guards attempt to calm him verbally or come too close, he strikes out.

You are asked to develop a treatment plan for the aggressive behavior, and you systematically consider the six sets of factors.

Medical Conditions: You wonder if Daniel's bathroom behavior is related to constipation. Because Daniel is nonverbal, your review of systems is adapted accordingly. You point to different body parts and ask "Pain? Hurts?" He shakes his head no to all body parts except to his abdomen. You request a gastrointestinal consult to rule out impaction/constipation or other problems. A flat plate of the abdomen shows evidence of impaction. Appropriate treatment is started, and his unusual bathroom behaviors diminish. You wonder whether those behaviors were not in fact a threat but, rather, a request for help with toileting due to the constipation.

You also observe that Daniel has a large head and low-set ears. You request a genetics consult, and a chromosome analysis, microarray, and whole exome sequencing are ordered. The results do not suggest any anomalies that could help explain his aggressive behavior.

Functional Communication Impairment: You recall wondering if Daniel can read. You call his school teacher and learn that he can read at a fifth-grade level and copy sentences. This indicates that Daniel had more means to communicate than is evident on casual observation. You ask that staff communicate with him in writing whenever possible and minimize verbal interactions (questions and complex explanations) that overwhelm Daniel's limited receptive and expressive spoken language abilities.

Psychosocial Stressors: The fact that Daniel did not show aggression in school is a major clue that the environment plays some role in his behavior. His teacher tells you that he seems to enjoy his school day, which is highly structured with many visual reminders of his schedule. He is always told in writing of a planned transition at least 10 minutes beforehand. Neither his grandparents nor the psychiatric inpatient unit were able to provide this predictability, and in both these settings irritability and aggressive behavior were frequent. You work with the team to approximate the consistency of the classroom within the constraints of the inpatient unit.

Maladaptive Reinforcement Patterns: Daniel's teacher tells you that Daniel will work for rewards, especially when the reward is access to a preferred activity such as a computer. Unfortunately, his grandparents allowed him unlimited, unconditional access to his computer at home. He had also learned that at home he could avoid activities that were sensorily aversive to him (e.g., showering) by showing aggression. You work with the inpatient staff to restructure access to the computer so it becomes a reward for keeping his hands down. You request a behavioral consultant to provide a plan for desensitizing Daniel to water and hope that he can continue the plan at his next placement.

Psychiatric Disorders: Based on further history and observations from the grandparents, teacher, and unit staff as well as the use of pictures with Daniel, you find no evidence for ADHD; an anxiety, mood, or obsessive–compulsive disorder; psychosis; or catatonia.

Irritability and Aggression Associated with Autism Spectrum Disorder: After systematic review of the other contributing factors, you conclude that his aggression both at home and on the inpatient unit is primarily related to irritability provoked by challenges to his core symptoms of ASD (insistence on sameness and sensory hypersensitivity).

The team has addressed the relevant medical, communication, psychosocial, and reinforcement concerns. Nonetheless, Daniel continues to have aggression around transitions and showering on the inpatient unit. For his safety and that of others, you elect to start Daniel on risperidone.

### Clinical Pearl

Sometimes, the severity of the aggression and/or environmental constraints will require emergency or ongoing intervention with psychotropic medications, such as neuroleptics. The US Food and Drug Administration has approved two medications, risperidone and aripiprazole, for the treatment of "irritability and aggression associated with autism." In a meta-analysis, Fung et al. (2016) found that risperidone and aripiprazole were effective. Individual studies with small sample sizes suggest that valproate and *N*-acetylcysteine may lead to improvements in Aberrant Behavior Checklist Irritability scale (ABC-I). In studies targeting hyperactivity as the primary outcome measure, clonidine, methylphenidate, and atomoxetine also resulted in improvements in ABC-I, although these studies were specifically performed in children with ASD and significant hyperactivity. Providing parent training is effective for improving behavior and adaptive functioning as well (Bearss et al., 2015).

Using national Medicaid claims, Mandell et al. (2008) found substantial psychotropic medication use among children with ASD, with 56% taking at least one psychotropic medication and 20% taking three or more medications. Among 18- to 21-year-olds with ASD, 49% were on neuroleptics. These high utilization rates speak to the importance of seeking other approaches to treating aggression in people with developmental disabilities. United States federal and state laws require review and approval of medication treatment for people with developmental disabilities, usually by community-based "human rights committees," as a safeguard in the absence of informed consent.

The inpatient team contacted the board of education and the office for the developmentally disabled. Because Daniel was still in school and younger than age 21, the board of education had started searching for residential facilities for him. After 2 months of a combined ED and inpatient unit stay, Daniel's aggression abated and he was transferred to a therapeutic residential school. How his grandparents continue to remain involved in his care remains to be seen. When he turns 21 years old, he will need to be transferred to a residential setting for adults with developmental disabilities. This itself will represent another complicated and difficult transition for both Daniel and the systems of care supporting him.

**Clinical Pearl**

Special education services in the United States are supported under the Individuals with Disabilities Education Act, which entitles children with disabilities to a free, appropriate public education in the least restrictive environment until 21 years of age. This federal law is discussed in further detail in Chapter 9.

Special education options range from least restrictive (e.g., special education services integrated into a general education classroom) to most restrictive (e.g., residential school). Common types of special education settings include small special education classrooms within a general education school or a self-contained special education school.

## DISCUSSION

### Systems of Care

The emotional costs of developmental disabilities such as ASD at an individual, family, and societal level are extremely high. Quality of life for persons with ASD has been shown to decline with age (Lubetsky, Handen, Lubetsky, & McGonigle,

2014). Medicaid Home and Community-Based Service (HCBS) waivers permit individuals with disabilities, whose families would not meet Medicaid eligibility criteria, to obtain Medicaid supported services. These services are broad and may include applied behavioral analysis, supports in the home (e.g., respite and community habilitation worker), and special supplies (e.g., communication boards). In adulthood, HCBS may cover day treatment programs and residential homes. Medicaid pays for the largest percentage of services for children with ASD nationally (Leslie et al., 2017).

The optimal organization of services for persons with developmental disabilities is an area of active discussion and controversy. The Medical Home model has been advanced as means of providing "coordinated, accessible, continuous, culturally competent care, screening, education, referrals, and follow up" (Lubetsky et al., 2014, p. 99). The Medical Home could be located in a primary care or behavioral health setting. Fueyo, Caldwell, Mattern, Zahid, and Foley (2015) have argued that the ongoing social, behavioral, and emotional issues of persons with ASD are better addressed in a center in which psychiatric expertise can be concentrated. However, for the vast majority of persons with developmental disabilities, the issue is not where to get care but, rather, how to get care at all. Access to care is limited by cost and insurance coverage, as well as lack of availability of providers who are willing to provide care to individuals with ASD (Liu, Pearl, Kong, Leslie, & Murray, 2017). This underscores the importance of training all medical and behavioral health providers to be comfortable with providing care for this population.

Due to limited outpatient services, persons with developmental disabilities may instead present to EDs and inpatient units for problem behaviors. The increase in adolescents with ASD presenting to an ED, from 3.1% in 2005 to 15.8% in 2013, is thought to reflect a deficit in services; ED use for non-ASD adolescents remained the same (approximately 3%) (Liu et al., 2017). Lunsky, Paquette-Smith, Weiss, and Lee (2015) found that adolescents with a history of aggressive behavior and a lack of structured daytime activities predicted higher rates of ED utilization by adolescents and adults with ASD. Some programs attempt to address this issue by offering community-based crisis and linkage services (see http://www.centerforstartservices.org).

"Psychiatric boarding," in which patients wait for an inpatient bed in the ED or on a medical unit, is a growing problem and may be related to the decrease in inpatient psychiatry beds nationally. Children with ASD, intellectual disability, and/or developmental delay are 2.5 times more likely to be boarded than typically developing children (Wharff, Ginnis, Ross, & Blood, 2011). Emergency departments often struggle to provide optimal care due to lack of knowledge about social services, time constraints to obtain needed information about the patient, and poor communication across agencies/services (Lunsky, Gracey, & Gelfand, 2008).

Despite these challenges, research is blossoming, early treatments are becoming more nuanced and widely available. Clinicians are becoming more specific in their diagnosis and treatment planning. Many more persons with developmental disabilities are living in the community and thriving there than a generation ago.

## ACKNOWLEDGMENTS

This work was supported by Marilyn and James Simon Family Giving through its support of the Whitaker Scholar Program in Developmental Neuropsychiatry at Columbia University. We thank Jeremy Veenstra-Vanderweele, MD, for his helpful comments.

## REFERENCES

American Psychiatric Association. (2013). *Diagnostic and statistical manual of mental disorders* (5th ed.). Arlington, VA: American Psychiatric Publishing.

Bearss, K., Johnson, C., Smith, T., Lecavalier, L., Swiezy, N., Aman, M., . . . Scahill, L. (2015). Effect of parent training vs. parent education on behavioral problems in children with autism spectrum disorder: A randomized clinical trial. *JAMA*, *313*(15), 1524–1533.

Fueyo, M., Caldwell, T., Mattern, S. B., Zahid, J., & Foley, T. (2015). The health home: A service delivery model for autism and intellectual disability. *Psychiatric Services*, *66*(11), 1135–1137. doi:10.1176/appi.ps.201400443

Fung, L. K., Mahajan, R., Nozzolillo, A., Bernal, P., Krasner, A., Jo, B., . . . Hardan, A. Y. (2016). Pharmacologic treatment of severe irritability and problem behaviors in autism: A systematic review and meta-analysis. *Pediatrics*, *137*(Suppl. 2), S124–S135. doi:10.1542/peds.2015-2851K

Leslie, D. L., Iskandarani, K., Dick, A. W., Mandell, D. S., Yu, H., Velott, D., . . . Stein, B. D. (2017). The effects of Medicaid home and community-based services waivers on unmet needs among children with autism spectrum disorder. *Medical Care*, *55*(1), 57–63. doi:10.1097/MLR.0000000000000621

Liu, G., Pearl, A. M., Kong, L., Leslie, D. L., & Murray, M. J. (2017). A profile on emergency department utilization in adolescents and young adults with autism spectrum disorders. *Journal of Autism and Developmental Disorders*, *47*(2), 347–358. doi:10.1007/s10803-016-2953-8

Lubetsky, M. J., Handen, B. L., Lubetsky, M., & McGonigle, J. J. (2014). Systems of care for individuals with autism spectrum disorder and serious behavioral disturbance through the lifespan. *Child and Adolescent Psychiatric Clinics of North America*, *23*(1), 97–110. doi:10.1016/j.chc.2013.08.004

Lunsky, Y., Gracey, C., & Gelfand, S. (2008). Emergency psychiatric services for individuals with intellectual disabilities: Perspectives of hospital staff. *Intellectual and Developmental Disabilities*, *46*(6), 446–455. doi:10.1352/2008.46:446–455

Lunsky, Y., Paquette-Smith, M., Weiss, J. A., & Lee, J. (2015). Predictors of emergency service use in adolescents and adults with autism spectrum disorder living with family. *Emergency Medicine Journal*, *32*(10), 787–792. doi:10.1136/emermed-2014-204015

Lyall, K., Croen, L., Daniels, J., Fallin, M. D., Ladd-Acosta, C., Lee, B. K., . . . Newschaffer, C. (2017). The changing epidemiology of autism spectrum disorders. *Annual Review of Public Health*, *38*, 81–102. doi:10.1146/annurev-publhealth-031816-044318

Mandell, D. S., Morales, K. H., Marcus, S. C., Stahmer, A. C., Doshi, J., & Polsky, D. E. (2008). Psychotropic medication use among Medicaid-enrolled children with autism spectrum disorders. *Pediatrics*, *121*(3), e441–e448. doi:10.1542/peds.2007-0984

McGuire, K., Fung, L. K., Hagopian, L., Vasa, R. A., Mahajan, R., Bernal, P., . . .
    Whitaker, A. H. (2016). Irritability and problem behavior in autism spectrum dis-
    order: A practice pathway for pediatric primary care. *Pediatrics*, *137*(Suppl. 2),
    S136–S148. doi:10.1542/peds.2015-2851L

Murphy, C. M., Wilson, C. E., Robertson, D. M., Ecker, C., Daly, E. M., Hammond,
    N., . . . McAlonan, G. M. (2016). Autism spectrum disorder in adults: Diagnosis,
    management, and health services development. *Neuropsychiatric Disease and
    Treatment*, *12*, 1669–1686. doi:10.2147/NDT.S65455

Wharff, E. A., Ginnis, K. B., Ross, A. M., & Blood, E. A. (2011). Predictors of
    psychiatric boarding in the pediatric emergency department: Implications
    for emergency care. *Pediatric Emergency Care*, *27*(6), 483–489. doi:10.1097/
    PEC.0b013e31821d8571

Wodka, E. L., Mathy, P., & Kalb, L. (2013). Predictors of phrase and fluent speech in
    children with autism and severe language delay. *Pediatrics*, *131*(4), e1128–e1134.

# 22

# HIV Psychiatry

**SHANE S. SPICER** ■

## CASE HISTORY

Mr. Michael Smith is a 26-year-old gay-identified African American cisgender man who is recently unemployed, newly single, and living in a homeless shelter near your inner-city community psychiatric clinic. Until 2 years ago, he was employed as a successful professional. He was referred to your clinic after being seen in the local emergency department 2 weeks ago. At the intake, he describes feeling sad and overwhelmed. He is experiencing tearfulness, hopelessness, low motivation, insomnia, ideas of reference, and vague paranoia. He is preoccupied with the fact that he was recently exposed to HIV during a sexual encounter. Although he has a long history of brief psychiatric hospitalizations, he is neither currently taking any psychotropic medications nor engaged in ongoing mental health treatment. He has never been engaged in primary care.

### Clinical Pearl

More than 1.1 million people in the United States are living with HIV infection, and almost 1 in 7 are unaware of their infection. Gay, bisexual, and other men who have sex with men (MSM), particularly young black/African American MSM, are most seriously affected by HIV (US Department of Health and Human Services, 2015).

Every patient encounter, whether in a medical or mental health setting, is a potential portal of entry for engagement and assessment of HIV, mental illness, and substance use disorders. Identification, prevention, and treatment of these comorbid illnesses greatly improve health outcomes.

When Mr. Smith reported his recent high-risk sexual behavior to the physician in the emergency department 2 weeks ago, he was offered a course of treatment with HIV post-exposure prophylaxis (PEP), sometimes known specifically as non-occupational HIV post-exposure prophylaxis (nPEP). Although Mr. Smith initiated treatment with PEP to potentially prevent acquiring HIV infection, he remains very worried about his health. He is currently adherent to the three antiretroviral medications (ARVs) prescribed, but he states that he has forgotten to take the medications on a few occasions due to his depression and the disorganized living situation in the shelter. He also has considered selling the ARVs to someone in his shelter in order to mitigate some of his financial stress.

### Clinical Pearl

Mental health care providers are frequently the first people who are contacted after a high-risk HIV exposure. Often, people are in great distress and need supportive counseling and concrete referrals during these crises. Therefore, psychiatrists should be aware of when PEP is indicated and be familiar with the referral procedures to the emergency department or other appropriate PEP providers in their communities.

According to the Centers for Disease Control and Prevention (CDC; 2016) and the New York State Department of Health AIDS Institute (2015b), PEP is proven to help prevent HIV infection after exposure to the virus. Exposure to HIV is a medical emergency. PEP should ideally be initiated within 2 hours and no later than 36 hours after exposure. However, it is sometimes initiated within 72 hours of exposure. The efficacy of PEP diminishes with delayed initiation. PEP includes a combination of antiretrovirals and should be taken consistently as prescribed, typically for 28 days. PEP can consist of various combinations of different ARVs depending on the clinical situation; therefore, checking for specific drug–drug interactions with other medications is advisable. Adherence is very important, and psychiatrists can be a source of support by problem-solving potential barriers to treatment adherence, including by managing the symptoms of mental illnesses. HIV testing should be offered by the PEP prescriber at baseline and at 4 and 12 weeks. A negative test at 12 weeks generally excludes HIV infection related to the exposure.

PEP is recommended for the following types of exposures:

- Condom-free receptive and insertive vaginal or anal intercourse with a person known to be HIV positive or whose HIV status is unknown
- Needle sharing
- Injuries with exposure to blood or other potentially infected fluids from a source known to be HIV infected or HIV status unknown

Upon gathering more history, Mr. Smith states that he originally brought himself to the emergency department 2 weeks ago due to racing thoughts, auditory hallucinations, and concerns that he was being monitored by a government agency through his cell phone. He also was having intense anxiety, intermittent panic attacks, and rumination that he had contracted a treatment-resistant strain of HIV. He had used intravenous crystal methamphetamine ("meth") for the 4 days prior to his emergency department visit. Typical of his binges on crystal meth for the past several years, he was using the substance to "PnP" or "party and play". He describes this as meeting anonymous men using online apps with whom to use "Tina" (crystal meth) and have "bareback" or "raw" (condom-free) anal sex. He states that his recent visit to the emergency department is just 1 of approximately 10 similar visits during the past year. He says that he has also been treated with PEP several times during the past year. He was first introduced to smoking crystal meth approximately 4 years ago by a friend, and his use has escalated in frequency and amount during the past 2 years. He states that he no longer smokes crystal meth but now exclusively "slams" (uses crystal meth intravenously).

## Clinical Pearl

Often, patients with comorbid HIV and psychiatric and substance use disorders (frequently referred to as "triple diagnosis") present a complex clinical picture. HIV and substance use can cause symptoms identical to those of almost any psychiatric illness, and with untreated comorbidities and complicating psychosocial stressors, diagnoses often remain provisional.

There is an ongoing public health crisis with methamphetamine use disorder in urban MSM communities that continues to fuel today's HIV crisis. Methamphetamine use disorder is often comorbid with depressive disorders, anxiety disorders, and post-traumatic stress disorder (PTSD). Crystal meth is very disinhibiting and is often used in the context of sex to help overcome shame and anxiety related to internalized homophobia/transphobia and difficulties with intimacy.

Patients are frequently misdiagnosed with primary psychotic disorders or bipolar disorders due to methamphetamine-induced psychotic and mood symptoms. Generally, these substance-induced symptoms subside within the first week of abstinence but can sometime persist for weeks or longer. Antipsychotic medications can be useful in these situations.

Records and lab results are requested from the emergency department where Mr. Smith had his initial crisis intervention. They include a normal brain computed tomography scan, lab results and physical exam, and a urine toxicology positive for methamphetamine. At your clinic, Mr. Smith is prescribed a low dose of an atypical antipsychotic at bedtime to help address mood symptoms, psychosis, and insomnia. He also agrees ambivalently to engage in the substance use treatment program affiliated with your mental health clinic. During the first 2 weeks of treatment, he maintains abstinence from crystal meth and finds support in the individual and group therapy offered. This is the first time he has engaged in consistent treatment, and he states that what has made this experience different is that the clinic is lesbian, gay, bisexual, transgender, and queer (LGBTQ)-affirmative and that there are other gay men in his groups with whom he can relate.

After Mr. Smith receives 2 weeks of treatment with the antipsychotic medication, the psychosis resolves. He continues to experience depressed mood, low energy, low motivation, and slowed cognition. Upon having a family meeting with his close friends and ex-partner, it is clarified that Mr. Smith has had manic and psychotic symptoms only in the context of active substance use but that he does have a long history of depressive symptoms predating his substance use disorder. He is interested in medication treatment to manage his current symptoms.

## Clinical Pearl

In general, when choosing psychotropic medications for people living with HIV/AIDS (PLWHA), use the following guidelines:

1. Doses: Start low and go slow.
2. If possible, avoid using multiple medications.
3. Remove unnecessary medications.
4. Check routinely for potential drug interactions. Many ARVs and psychotropic medications share the same cytochrome P450 metabolic pathways.
5. When possible, avoid medications with toxicities.

Antidepressants are the most commonly prescribed class of psychotropic medications for PLWHA. Selective serotonin reuptake inhibitors, particularly citalopram and escitalopram, are frequently preferred because they have less potential for drug interactions with ARVs compared to other antidepressants (Hill & Lee, 2013).

Some antidepressants can play a dual role in the treatment of PLWHA. For example, duloxetine may help with neuropathic pain caused by HIV/AIDS and certain ARVs; mirtazipine can increase appetite in PLWHA who have difficulty maintaining adequate weight (McDaniel et al., 2010); and bupropion can improve energy, motivation, and concentration, which can be impacted by both HIV and crystal meth use. However, currently, no pharmacologic agents are conclusively effective in treating methamphetamine use disorder (Heinzerling et al., 2014; Karila et al., 2010).

Little research has specifically examined antipsychotic use in this population. PLWHA have higher rates of extrapyramidal side effects, so atypical antipsychotics may be preferred, but the potential for metabolic side effects requires shared decision-making and monitoring (Hill & Lee, 2013).

After resolution of the methamphetamine-induced psychotic and mood symptoms, the atypical antipsychotic medication is discontinued. Mr. Smith is now started on bupropion for the treatment of depression. He responds well and is linked to housing and career development resources. He remains reluctant to go for his follow-up HIV testing. At each point of contact, the staff discuss with him the benefits of HIV testing and, if negative, the potential option of initiating HIV pre-exposure prophylaxis (PrEP). There is also ongoing education about the benefits of treating HIV, the successful outcomes of treatment, and exploring what being diagnosed with HIV would mean to him and how you could help him manage this diagnosis. It is also recommended that he be tested for hepatitis C given his history of intravenous drug use.

Staff use ongoing motivational interviewing regarding medical follow-up and safer sex practices, including the use of condoms. He processes the idea of HIV and hepatitis C testing with other clients in his substance use treatment groups and, with their support, decides to proceed. He agrees to see a primary care physician who works on-site at your clinic 2 days per week to further discuss PrEP. He schedules and attends the appointment, is found to be both HIV and hepatitis C negative, and is advised to discontinue PEP treatment. When you meet at your most recent psychiatric follow-up appointment, his other lab results are pending and he is awaiting a follow-up appointment with his new primary care doctor to further discuss PrEP. Although overwhelmed by his current life situation, he is feeling connected to others, optimistic, and more empowered and interested in his health and future goals.

## Clinical Pearl

According to the CDC (2015) and the New York State Department of Health AIDS Institute (2015a), PrEP is a way for people who do not have HIV infection, but who are at substantial risk of contracting it, to prevent HIV infection by taking a pill every day. The pill (brand name Truvada) currently approved for PrEP is taken once daily and is a combination of two medicines (tenofovir and emtricitabine). When someone is exposed to HIV through sex or injection drug use, this medication can work to keep the virus from establishing a permanent infection. When taken consistently, it can reduce the risk of HIV infection in people who are at high risk by up to 92%–99%. It is much less effective if not taken consistently.

Typically, an individual will be asked to see their doctor again after the first month of treatment, then at least every 3 months, for lab monitoring including kidney function, sexually transmitted illness (STI) testing, hepatitis infection testing, and HIV testing. Also, at follow-ups, clients should be given ongoing education about using condoms and that PrEP does not protect against any other STIs. Absolute contraindications are documented HIV infection, creatinine clearance less than 60 mL/min, and unreadiness to adhere to treatment. Nephrotoxic medications, such as lithium, should be avoided with Truvada, if possible.

Potential candidates for PrEP are non-HIV-infected individuals in the following groups:

- MSM who engage in condom-free anal intercourse
- Individuals who are in a serodiscordant sexual relationship with a known HIV-infected partner
- Transgender individuals engaging in high-risk sexual behaviors
- Individuals engaging in transactional sex, such as sex for money, drugs, or housing: This can occur among people with unstable economic and housing situations and people with serious mental illness (SMI).
- People who inject drugs and engage in high-risk behaviors such as needle sharing
- Individuals who use stimulant drugs associated with high-risk behaviors, such as methamphetamine
- Individuals diagnosed with at least one anogenital sexually transmitted infection in the past year
- Individuals who have been prescribed nPEP who demonstrate continued high-risk behavior or have used multiple courses of nPEP

## DISCUSSION

There are complex, interacting biological, psychological, and social relationships among mental illnesses, substance use disorders, and the HIV epidemic. They are syndemic, and without managing each, the HIV epidemic will not be adequately controlled and people with mental illness and substance use disorders will remain vulnerable to HIV infection.

The majority of PLWHA will have a diagnosable mental illness (Stoff, Mitnick, & Kalichman, 2004). Mental illnesses in this population can occur in many contexts.

They can be a risk factor for HIV infection, a psychological response to HIV infection, a result of the direct effect of HIV on the brain, a consequence of HIV-related opportunistic infections, and a side effect of HIV-related treatments. Depression and anxiety disorders are the most common mental illnesses in PLWHA and are as much as 5–10 times more prevalent than in the general US population. Lifetime prevalence of PTSD, alcohol use disorders, and other substance use disorders is significantly higher in PLWHA than in the general US population (Joska, Stein, & Grant, 2014). Some studies show suicide rates up to 3 times higher in PLWHA than in the general US population (Carrico, 2010; Keiser et al., 2010).

Untreated mental illness is associated with HIV-related risk-taking behaviors, transmission of HIV and other STIs, impaired ability to cope with HIV diagnosis, poorer HIV prognosis, less access to HIV treatment, decreased treatment adherence, diminished quality of life, increased health care costs, and higher mortality (Joska et al., 2014). "Triple diagnosis" carries a particular risk for decreased HIV viral suppression (Soto, Bell, & Pillen, 2004).

People with SMI are a population that is often unrecognized as being at high risk for HIV infection. Studies have found seroprevalence rates ranging from 3% to 23%, and people with SMI have been found to have the following risk behaviors: multiple sexual partners, unprotected intercourse, and injection drug use (Meade & Sikkema, 2005). Symptoms such as impulsivity, disinhibition, and poor judgment can place these individuals in risky situations. Also, persons with an SMI are more likely to live in risky environments; experience sexual coercion and intimate partner violence; have unstable partnerships in high-risk sexual networks; use substances that can impair decision-making; and lack the emotional stability, judgment, and interpersonal skills needed to avoid risks (Carey, Carey, & Kalichman, 1997).

During the past few decades, HIV has become more of a chronic illness due to better treatments. Acute neuropsychiatric presentations such as psychosis and mania are now less common, whereas subacute neurocognitive deficits are more prevalent. Even with undetectable viral loads, the central nervous system (CNS) can act as a reservoir for HIV. Some data suggest that using ARVs with better blood–brain barrier penetration can better decrease CNS infection and sequelae. The effects of HIV in the CNS are thought to be related to neurotoxic and inflammatory processes. There is evidence that this process can be further exacerbated by comorbid methamphetamine use as well as hepatitis C co-infection (Chana et al., 2006; Cherner et al., 2005).

Organizational models that have proven most effective for the treatment of PLWHA with behavioral health needs are those that offer integrated, co-located services. Ideally, the clinic would be located within a convenient and welcoming neighborhood for the clients being served and offer a "one-stop" model where people are able to receive medical, psychiatric, and substance use treatment, as well as case management and other support services. Where co-location is not possible, care managers can facilitate coordination in a busy community health care environment. A sensitive, trauma-informed treatment approach can improve engagement, retention, and adherence to care. Housing support, occupational resources, and other "wrap-around" services can prevent and eliminate barriers to care. Furthermore, community-specific groups and programs can increase connections in marginalized communities and support access to care.

From a public health standpoint, as described by the CDC, the National Institutes of Health, and the World Health Organization, there are several strategies being employed to address the HIV epidemic: prevention, testing, and treatment. Treatment as prevention (TasP) aims to engage people in ARV treatment at all stages of diagnosis and to provide necessary supports to increase adherence and promote viral suppression, with the goal of decreasing individual and community viral load and preventing risk of HIV transmission. Public psychiatrists can provide leadership and advocacy to promote TasP and integrate services in the battle against the HIV epidemic.

## REFERENCES

Carey, M. P., Carey, K. B., & Kalichman, S. C. (1997). Risk for human immunodeficiency virus (HIV) infection among persons with severe mental illnesses. *Clinical Psychology Review, 17*(3), 271–291.

Carrico, A. (2010). Elevated suicide rate among HIV-positive persons despite benefits of antiretroviral therapy: Implications for a stress and coping model of suicide. *American Journal of Psychiatry, 167*(2), 117–119.

Centers for Disease Control and Prevention. (2015). *Pre-exposure prophylaxis (PrEP).* Retrieved from https://www.cdc.gov/hiv/risk/prep/. Accessed July 1, 2017.

Centers for Disease Control and Prevention. (2016). Updated guidelines for antiretroviral postexposure prophylaxis after sexual, injection drug use, or other nonoccupational exposure to HIV—United States, 2016. Retrieved from https://www.cdc.gov/hiv/risk/pep/. Accessed July 1, 2017.

Chana, G., Everall, I. P., Crews, L., Langford, D., Adame, A., Grant, I., . . . Ellis, R.; the HNRC Group. (2006). Cognitive deficits and degeneration of interneurons in HIV+ methamphetamine users. *Neurology, 67*(8), 1486–1489.

Cherner, M., Letendre, S., Heaton, R. K., Durelle, J., Marquie-Beck, J., Gragg, B., & Grant, I.; the HNRC Group. (2005). Hepatitis C augments cognitive deficits associated with HIV infection and methamphetamine. *Neurology, 64*(8), 1343–1347.

Heinzerling, K. G., Swanson, A. N., Hall, T. M., Yi, Y., Wu, Y., & Shoptaw, S. J. (2014). Randomized, placebo-controlled trial of bupropion in methamphetamine-dependent participants with less than daily methamphetamine use. *Addiction, 109*(11), 1878–1886.

Hill, L., & Lee, K. C. (2013). Pharmacotherapy considerations in patients with HIV and psychiatric disorders: Focus on antidepressants and antipsychotics. *Annals of Pharmacotherapy, 47*, 75–89.

Joska, J. A., Stein, D. J., & Grant, I. (2014). *HIV and psychiatry.* West Sussex, UK: Wiley.

Karila, L., Weinstein, A., Aubin, H., Benyamina, A., Reynaud, M., & Batki, S. (2010). Pharmacological approaches to methamphetamine dependence: A focused review. *British Journal of Clinical Pharmacology, 69*(6), 578–592.

Keiser, O., Spoerri, A., Brinkhoff, M. W., Hasse, B., Gayet-Ageron, A., Tissot, F., . . . Egger, M. (2010). Suicide in HIV-infected individuals and the general population in Switzerland, 1988–2008. *American Journal of Psychiatry, 167*(2), 143–150.

McDaniel, J. S., Brown, L., Cournos, F., Forstein, M., Goodkin, K., Lykestos, C., & Chung, J. Y.; Work Group on HIV/AIDS. (2010). *Practice guidelines for the treatment of patients with HIV/AIDS.* Retrieved from http://psychiatryonline.org/pb/

assets/raw/sitewide/practice_guidelines/guidelines/hivaids.pdf. Accessed July 1, 2017.

Meade, C. S., & Sikkema, K. J. (2005). HIV risk behavior among adults with severe mental illness: A systematic review. *Clinical Psychology Review, 25*(4), 433–457.

New York State Department of Health AIDS Institute. (2015a). *Guidance for the use of PrEP.* Retrieved from http://www.hivguidelines.org/prep-for-prevention/. Accessed July 1, 2017.

New York State Department of Health AIDS Institute. (2015b). *PEP for non-occupational exposure to HIV guideline.* Retrieved from http://www.hivguidelines.org/pep-for-hiv-prevention/. Accessed July 1, 2017.

Soto, T. A., Bell, J., & Pillen, M. B. (2004). Literature on integrated HIV care: A review. *AIDS Care, 16*(1 Suppl.), S43–S55.

Stoff, D. M., Mitnick, L., & Kalichman, S. (2004). Research issues in the multiple diagnoses of HIV/AIDS, mental illness and substance abuse. *AIDS Care, 16*(1 Suppl.), S1–S5.

US Department of Health and Human Services. (2015). *U.S. statistics.* Retrieved from https://www.hiv.gov/hiv-basics/overview/data-and-trends/statistics. Accessed July 1, 2017.

# 23

# Refugees and Immigrants

POH CHOO HOW,\* PACHIDA LO,\*
MARJORIE WESTERVELT, AND HENDRY TON ■

## CASE HISTORY

Ms. Xiong is a 56-year-old Hmong woman referred to your clinic by her primary care provider for depression. Ms. Xiong is a monolingual Hmong speaker. In the initial intake, the social worker utilized her daughter as an interpreter. Ms. Xiong and her daughter felt uncomfortable with this arrangement, but they agreed to participate. She denied feeling depressed, but she complained of body aches and insomnia that significantly impacted her ability to care for her children and household. She presents to you for a psychiatric assessment.

### Clinical Pearl

Patients with limited English proficiency experience more communication challenges, which can result in worse outcomes (Divi, Koss, Schmaltz, & Loeb, 2007). Therefore, trained interpreters are crucial in these contexts. The use of family members or untrained staff can lead to misinterpretation and confidentiality problems. In mental health settings, in which sensitive information may arise, untrained interpreters may be uncomfortable communicating potentially embarrassing information (Ton & Lim, 2015). If an in-person interpreter is not available, telephone interpreters may be used. Interpreters with cultural knowledge can also serve as cultural brokers and provide cultural interpretation, conveying not only the patient's statements but also the cultural context to more accurately reflect the patient's experience.

In your clinic, you are fortunate to work with a trained interpreter. To help inform how you will approach the interview, you ask the interpreter to arrive early to review how depression is commonly perceived and discussed within Ms. Xiong's culture.
  Ms. Xiong is encouraged to talk about her health beliefs concerning her mood and physical ailments. She reports that none of the antidepressants previously

\* Co-first authors.

prescribed have helped with her pain and stress. The pharmacist informed her that the information leaflet for her medication stated that it was for "crazy people." She does not believe that she is "crazy," and so she rarely takes her medications. Ms. Xiong reports not understanding the need to take daily medications. She feared telling doctors about her nonadherence due to fear of retribution and losing other forms of social support, especially disability benefits. She states that she is beginning to lose hope of getting better. She considered consulting a shaman to determine the cause of her symptoms but is unable to afford one. Instead, she takes traditional herbal treatments for her pain and stress.

## Clinical Pearl

Perspectives about mental illness, its expression, and treatments often differ significantly between immigrants/refugees and their providers. These differences contribute to misunderstandings and unexpressed disagreements that negatively impact the treatment process. Addressing these cultural differences using face-saving communication is critical to minimize stigma and feelings of shame. For example, providers should consider exploring somatic complaints before emotional ones (Fancher, Ton, Le Meyer, Ho, & Paterniti, 2010). Another important step is to elicit the patient's explanatory model (Figure 23.1) and emphasize areas of provider–patient agreement.

Providers should discuss the patient's beliefs about the causes, symptoms, and impact of his or her illness. Once that has been established, the next step is to gauge the patient's preferred mode of treatment and overall treatment goals. Consider also that patients who are collectivistically oriented may not

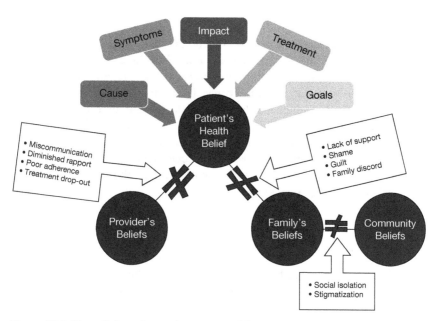

Figure 23.1 The collaborative explanatory model.

feel comfortable following through with treatment decisions unless they consult with their families.

According to Ms. Xiong's explanatory model, many of her health beliefs are grounded in her spirituality. She reports concern about her spirit being lost as a cause of her pain, low energy, and poor sleep. Although there was disagreement regarding the cause and treatment between the providers and the patient, you establish an alliance based on your shared concern about her symptoms, their impact, and her treatment goals. You also facilitate involvement of a shaman of her choice in her treatment plan. (You are fortunate that traditional healing is budgeted as a line item at your clinic. Funding for this otherwise may come from the patient or kinship networks.) Finally, you establish that she prefers to have her children and husband help her make treatment decisions and therefore involve them in future visits. You consult with the family about incorporating shaman treatment while also starting her on a longer acting antidepressant, given her potential to miss doses. They approve of this plan and commit to helping her follow through. A month later, she reports improved sleep, energy, and appetite, although she continues to report feelings of demoralization and isolation given continued chronic pain.

As treatment progresses, Ms. Xiong becomes more comfortable talking about her past. She describes being born in Laos and fleeing with her family to a refugee camp in Thailand to escape the Secret War (Laotian Civil War). She married at the age of 15 and moved to Sacramento, California, in 1982 with her husband and three young children.

### Clinical Pearl

Significant risk factors and stressors exist during all phases of migration. These have long-lasting effects on mental health (see Table 23.1). Hence, providers should explore areas of trauma and loss in the migration history. Trauma can also trigger personal growth and reveal resilience. Resilience is conceptualized as a process involving dynamic interactions between risk and protective factors, internal (e.g., biology and personality) and external (e.g., social support) to a person at various stages. Some have conceptualized resilience as an adaptive process in which an individual has the the ability to transform trauma into positive personal growth experiences (Polk, 1997). This positive change after a traumatic experience is called *post-traumatic growth* (PTG). There are five major domains of PTG: personal strength, new possibilities, relating to others, appreciation of life, and spiritual change (Tedeschi & Calhoun, 1996).

Providers can foster resilience in individuals who have suffered from trauma by promoting environments that enable social cohesion. The provider can reinforce and build upon resilience factors, for example, by using strengths-based psychotherapy to facilitate connection with spirituality. Group therapy and community integration can also enhance mental health and overall development.

Ms. Xiong suffered tremendous loss and trauma relating to her migration. Separation from her family members significantly narrowed her support network. However, Ms. Xiong's personal strength and spirituality helped her cope with trauma. To further facilitate resilience and PTG, you work on addressing both her internal and her external resilience factors. You provide psychotherapy to foster the validation and growth of her personal strengths and spirituality that have enabled her to have the will to survive and overcome trauma. For external support, you provide her with transportation to engage her in social rehabilitation; assist her in obtaining US citizenship; and involve her in a support group for Hmong women, which over time appears to help her.

Ms. Xiong reports reduced hopelessness. She has also found greater meaning in spending time with her children and believes there is less importance to being attached to extrinsic items and "making lots of money."

## DISCUSSION

The number of refugees worldwide continues to increase, with an estimated 19.5 million in 2014, of which 69,000 resettled in the United States during that year alone (Martin & Yankay, 2014; United Nations High Commissioner for Refugees, 2015). In addition, in 2014, an estimated 11 million unauthorized immigrants were recorded to reside in the United States (Rosenblum & Ruiz Soto, 2015). There are unique differences between immigrants and refugees, including differences in mental health outcomes. An immigrant is a "voluntary" migrant who leaves his or her home country in hopes for a better life (Walker & Barnett, 2007). A refugee is a "forced" migrant "who is unable or unwilling to return to his or her country of nationality because of persecution or a well-founded fear of persecution on account of race, religion, nationality, membership in a particular social group, or political opinion" (Martin & Yankay, 2014, p. 1). Unlike immigrants, refugees are forced out of their country and unable to return. An asylum seeker is a refugee who is already in or at a port of entry seeking admittance into the host country. All three groups leave their home countries due to suboptimal living conditions and encounter similar challenges in the pre-migration, migration, and post-migration phases. Compared to immigrants, refugees are at a significantly higher risk for developing mental illness (Walker & Barnett, 2007).

Common mental health conditions among refugees and immigrants include: anxiety, depression, and somatization (Walker & Barnett, 2007). Some studies have found rates of post-traumatic stress disorder (PTSD) in Cambodian refugees as high as 50%, whereas rates of PTSD in Bosnian refugees ranged from 18% to 53% (Watters, 2001). There does seem to be a link between PTSD and major depressive disorder (MDD) across refugee and immigrant groups. It is noted that 71% of migrants with PTSD also met the diagnostic criteria for MDD; and, 86% of individuals with MDD met diagnostic criteria for PTSD (Walker & Barnett, 2007). This comorbidity is also linked to a higher likelihood of suicide, particularly in women (Walker & Barnett, 2007). Schizophrenia has also been found in higher rates in migrants who moved from developing to developed nations compared to individuals who remained in their host country (Walker & Barnett, 2007).

Treatment of mental illness in this population requires culturally sensitive approaches and attention to the specific stressors associated with being a migrant (Table 23.1). Resiliency factors that can affect an individual's treatment and recovery include the individual's sense of self-esteem or self-confidence, ability to cope with change, level of social problem-solving skills, and strength of self-identity (Watters, 2001).

*Table 23.1* Risk Factors Associated with Pre-migration, Migration, and Post-migration

| Stage of Migration | Stressors/Risk Factors for Mental Illness |
| --- | --- |
| Pre-migration (prior to leaving home country) | War, violence, torture, sexual abuse, loss of social, familial, and material resources |
| Migration (travel/placement before host country) | Prolonged refugee detention, forced versus voluntary migration, longer distances traveled, longer wait periods before asylum status granted, illegal immigration, intramigration trauma |
| Post-migration (resettlement) | Poor proficiency in the language of the host-country, lack of housing and employment, discrimination, difficulty adapting to local culture, separation from family or friends |

sources: Walker and Barnett (2007) and Watters (2001).

The level of acculturation with the host or dominant culture also affects immigrant and refugee mental health. Acculturation refers to the changes in identity, values, behavior, and attitudes that occur through contact with another culture (Berry, 1997). Different types of acculturation result from two basic issues that migrants have to consider: (1) the degree to which they affiliate with their own culture and (2) the degree to which they affiliate with the host culture (Table 23.2).

Marginalization occurs when one rejects his or her own culture but also does not adopt the majority culture. Assimilation occurs when one rejects his or her own culture and adopts the majority culture. Rejection of the dominant culture while maintaining one's original culture results in separation from the dominant culture. By contrast, maintaining one's values and cultural identity while simultaneously maintaining positive relations with the dominant group results in integration. Some studies have shown that groups that have achieved integration have more positive mental health outcomes (Rumbaut, 1991) and that marginalization is correlated with increased emotional distress among Third World immigrants in First World countries (Sam & Berry, 1995). Of the different acculturating groups, refugees are the most vulnerable to acculturative stress, with overall reduction in psychological, somatic, and social domains (Sam & Berry, 1995).

The general orientation of a host society toward immigrants and refugees and toward cultural pluralism plays an indelible role in the refugee experience of acculturation. Societies that support cultural pluralism will have a positive impact on

*Table 23.2* Fourfold Acculturation Model

| | | Degree of Affiliation with Original Culture | |
| --- | --- | --- | --- |
| | | High | Low |
| Degree of Affiliation with Host Culture | High | Integration | Assimilation |
| | Low | Separation (rejection) | Marginality (deculturation) |

source: Berry (1997).

refugee acculturation, whereas those that seek to eliminate diversity through policies and programs of assimilation further marginalize the population, contributing to psychological distress (Berry, 1997).

All refugees are required to undergo a health assessment upon arrival into the United States (Figure 23.2). This is coordinated by state-level refugee health programs and conducted in local health departments, community health centers, or private clinics. In addition to a general medical examination checklist, the Centers for Disease Control and Prevention (2014) has also published a set of guidelines to assess the mental health status of newly arrived refugees. All newly arrived refugees also receive assistance at the state level to apply for Medicaid benefits. Individuals who do not qualify for Medicaid benefits can receive federally funded health care coverage for up to 8 months through the Refugee Medical Assistance program. (Minnesota Department of Human Services, 2016).

For undocumented immigrants, the fear of being detained by immigration authorities is a barrier to seeking care at all or at least until symptoms are very severe. At the same time, welfare reform legislation prevents them from accessing federal programs such as Medicaid. There may be limited programs available in some states and counties (New York, Washington, DC, and some California

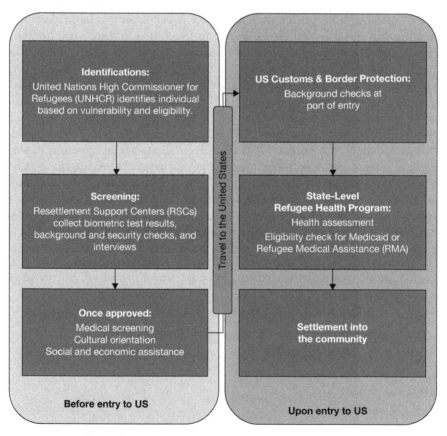

Figure 23.2 Pathway of a refugee into the United States.
SOURCE: US Citizenship and Immigration Services (2015).

counties), but access to care is usually limited to public, volunteer, and charitable clinics (Okie, 2007).

In the United States, several models of community-based mental health clinics and community health centers serve immigrant and refugees—for example, the Transcultural Wellness Center in Sacramento, California; the Intercultural Psychiatric Program at Oregon Health & Science University; and the University of Minnesota Community–University Health Care Center. Interdisciplinary collaboration among psychiatry, case management, interpreters, legal clinic and other primary care medical providers, and dentistry and pharmacy is key to these programs. They rely heavily on public funding and county support. The programs are often held to the same practice standards as mainstream providers in the counties that they serve; however, the reimbursement level is often low, which leads to financial challenges (Boehnlein et al., 2015).

Refugees and immigrants bring significant benefits of cultural diversity and economic vitality to their host countries. However, negative experiences during pre-, intra-, and post-migration may lead to greater psychological distress. Mental health providers should strive to (1) ensure effective communication through appropriate use of a trained interpreter when necessary, (2) develop a collaborative explanatory model that can serve as a common starting point for the healing process, (3) identify and foster resilience and post-traumatic growth, and (4) address socioeconomic factors that are barriers to adaptive acculturation and meaningful participation in community. Community mental health providers have an important role in the care for migrants given challenges with legal status, insurance, and poverty. Successful mental health treatment often involves embracing biopsychosocial approaches that integrate diverse sectors of support, including primary care providers, nonprofit agencies, social service agencies, policymakers, and faith-based organizations.

## REFERENCES

Berry, J. W. (1997). Immigration, acculturation, and adaptation. *Applied Psychology*, *46*(1), 5–34.

Boehnlein, J. K., Kinzie, J. D., Leung, P. K., Cary M., Cheng, K., & Sedighi, B. (2015). The intercultural psychiatric program at Oregon Health and Science University. In L. W. Roberts, D. Reicherter, S. Adelsheim, S. V. Joshi (Eds.), *Partnerships for Mental Health* (pp. 147–161). New York: Springer.

Centers for Disease Control and Prevention. (2014, May 8). Guidelines for mental health screening during the domestic medical examination for newly arrived refugees. *Immigrant and Refugee Health*. Retrieved from http://www.cdc.gov/immigrantrefugeehealth/guidelines/domestic/mental-health-screening-guidelines.html. Accessed November, 9, 2016.

Divi, C., Koss, R. G., Schmaltz, S. P., & Loeb, J. M. (2007). Language proficiency and adverse events in US hospitals: A pilot study. *International Journal for Quality in Health Care*, *19*(2), 60–67.

Fancher, T. L., Ton, H., Le Meyer, O., Ho, T., & Paterniti, D. A. (2010). Discussing depression with Vietnamese American patients. *Journal of Immigrant and Minority Health*, *12*(2), 263–266.

Martin, D. C., & Yankay, J. E. (2014). *Refugees and asylees 2013*. Retrieved from http://www.dhs.gov/publication/refugees-and-asylees-2013#

Minnesota Department of Human Services. (2016, June 1). Minnesota health care programs eligibility policy manual. *Refugee Medical Assistance (RMA)*. Retrieved from http://hcopub.dhs.state.mn.us/03_45_10.htm#Covered_heading. Accessed November 9, 2016.

Okie, S. (2007). Immigrants and health care – at the intersection of two broken systems. *New England Journal of Medicine*, 357(6), 525–529.

Polk, L. V. (1997). Toward a middle-range theory of resilience. *Advances in Nursing Science*, 19(3), 1–13.

Rosenblum, M. R., & Ruiz Soto, A. G. (2015). *An analysis of unauthorized immigrants in the United States by country and region of birth*. Washington, DC: Migration Policy Institute.

Rumbaut, R. G. (1991). Migration, adaptation, and mental health: The experience of Southeast Asian refugees in the United States. In H. Adelman (Ed.), *Refugee policy: Canada and the United States* (pp. 383–427). Toronto, Ontario, Canada: York Lanes Press.

Sam, D. L., & Berry, J. W. (1995). Acculturative stress among young immigrants in Norway. *Scandinavian Journal of Psychology*, 36(1), 10–24.

Tedeschi, R. G., & Calhoun, L. G. (1996). The Posttraumatic Growth Inventory: Measuring the positive legacy of trauma. *Journal of Traumatic Stress*, 9(3), 455–471.

Ton, H., & Lim, R. (2015). Assessment of culturally diverse individuals: Introduction and foundations. In R. F. Lim (Ed.), *Clinical manual of cultural psychiatry* (2 ed.). Washington, DC: American Psychiatric Publishing.

United Nations High Commissioner for Refugees. (2015). *Global trends: Forced displacement in 2014*. Geneva, Switzerland: Author.

US Citizenship and Immigration Services. (2015, December 3). *Refugee processing and security screening*. Retrieved from https://www.uscis.gov/refugeescreening#RefugeeProcessing. Accessed November 9, 2016.

Walker, P. F., & Barnett, E. D. (2007). *Immigrant medicine*. St. Louis, MO: Saunders/Elsevier.

Watters, C. (2001). Emerging paradigms in the mental health care of refugees. *Social Science & Medicine*, 52(11), 1709–1718.

# 24

# Rural Communities

RYAN P. PEIRSON AND PAULETTE MARIE GILLIG ■

## CASE HISTORY

Abby is a 28-year-old single mother of two who is seeing you for the first time for a chief complaint of anxiety. Working in a rural community mental health center, you are the first psychiatrist she has seen face to face in several years. She is currently taking alprazolam 2 mg PO TID as monotherapy for anxiety prescribed by a remote psychiatrist using telemedicine technology. She has been driving 2 hours to a larger town to see "a doctor on a video screen." Abby preferred to see you locally, but your availability kept her on a waiting list.

### Clinical Pearl: Telemedicine and Transportation Issues

Telemedicine, including telepsychiatry, is increasing dramatically in rural environments. Allowing access to providers otherwise unable or unwilling to travel to the areas in need, telepsychiatry can be a welcome solution to access woes. It is not available everywhere, and some people still have to travel long distances to see a telepsychiatrist. Just as people in rural environments can sometimes drive many miles to go shopping or to school, they may have to drive many miles to seek medical care. Lack of transportation is a major barrier to care in rural communities and a significant cause of missed appointments (Syed, Gerber, & Sharp, 2013).

When discussing her anxiety, you learn Abby has taken alprazolam for years. It was initially started at a lower dose as a temporary medication by her family doctor. Over time, the dose was slowly increased. Because it was helping, her family doctor was reluctant to try different medications. The telepsychiatrist suggested several medications that Abby could not obtain due to their cost. Although desperately concerned that she can afford nothing else that relieves her symptoms, Abby is genuinely open to trying other medications and is grateful for your suggestions. Because she has never taken fluoxetine and has no apparent contraindications, you suggest beginning a trial. She participates in a managed care plan through her state Medicaid benefit, which has a very narrow formulary. Concerned that her coverage might lapse, you confirm that the medication is on a list of less expensive generic medications that cost only $4.00 at her local grocery store.

### Clinical Pearl: Medication Choices

Although a federally administered program, Medicaid plans are ultimately managed by the states. Certain benefits are required, but factors such as eligibility, personal cost, and specific benefits can vary widely from state to state. Even within individual states, benefits may differ slightly from one person to another. Some states require participation in a managed care plan, and some allow for a measure of choice. Of course, commercial insurance plans can have major differences, and even with Medicare, individuals have different levels of coverage. Not necessarily an issue unique to rural areas, it should be noted that access, resources, and benefits are different from community to community. Not every pharmacy, clinic, or hospital has a contract with Medicaid or with every commercial insurance product. For those requiring treatment with an antipsychotic, long-acting injectable medications may add a measure of security. With regard to medication samples, depending on multiple factors, pharmaceutical representatives do not always call on rural clinics and samples may not be available. Major retail pharmacies and grocery chains have competitive pricing lists for generic medication, and this can be advantageous depending on their penetration into the rural markets.

Abby is able to identify several anxiety symptom triggers and can describe alleviating and exacerbating factors. You discuss this with her and decide that she might do well with a course of cognitive–behavioral therapy. Thinking it would be worth trying a planned 12-week program, you decide to consult with the therapist in your clinic who uses cognitive–behavioral therapy. Unfortunately, the therapist would only be able to see Abby one time per month due to the limited therapy hours available.

### Clinical Pearl: Access to Psychotherapy

Access to psychotherapy is correlated with living in a metropolitan area (Fortney, Harman, Xu, & Dong, 2009). The more rural the environment, the less likely a person will have access to psychotherapy at all, let alone high-quality psychotherapy.

You consider providing regular psychotherapy yourself. When checking your calendar, you remember that the community is heavily reliant on your ability to maintain access for medication management. You must sparingly commit to more frequent appointments lest you limit your availability for another patient to be seen. You realize it will not be possible for you to do psychotherapy with her at this time.

### Clinical Pearl: Billable Time

An aspect of public psychiatry that can be accentuated in rural psychiatry is administrative pressure for "billable time." Psychiatrist time is an expensive resource. Some practices or clinics can ill-afford professional services, and administrators apply significant pressure to "produce." When this occurs, it can be at the expense of almost anything other than billable face-to-face encounters with evaluation and management codes. This can make it more difficult for rural public psychiatrists to participate in leadership activities and team-based care.

Abby explains it is also difficult to find treatment for her back pain. She is concerned that her primary care physician will stop prescribing oxycodone and asks if you are willing to provide it for her. As you begin to discuss her substance use history, Abby states that she must rely on an old boyfriend for transportation. He is very demanding and often tries to manipulate her into giving him her prescription medications. She thinks he has stolen her oxycodone in the past.

### Clinical Pearl: Opioid Abuse in Rural Areas

Recently, rural nonmedical use of prescription opioids has been of particular concern. Rural users of illicit prescription opioids show differences in use patterns compared to urban counterparts. An increased incidence in use of other drugs in combination with opioids is observed, as is an earlier age of onset (Young, Havens, & Leukefeld, 2012). Rural users report using prescription oxycodone the most often among illicit substances (Young et al., 2012). Of note, overdose deaths related to illicit opioid use are often in the context of concurrent benzodiazepine use (Centers for Disease Control and Prevention, 2015).

Together with Abby, you search online for specialty outpatient substance treatment programs and learn, as you have come to expect, that Abby will have to travel 1 hour to participate, which will not be realistic given her reliance on her old boyfriend for transportation. Instead, the two of you, in collaboration with Abby's primary care physician, make a plan to taper and discontinue her opioids and benzodiazepines. During that 2-month period, you are able to see her every other week instead of once every 2 months. After another 2 months, Abby tells you with pride that she has been working with the clinic's case manager and, with her assistance, applied for a job at a local grocery store. Later in the month, while shopping, you are surprised to see Abby is the cashier. Despite your wise shopping choices, you become acutely aware of your ice cream indiscretions and the sundry, intimate, personal items you are loath to turn over to a stranger, let alone a patient. When it is your turn, Abby makes eye contact, smiles, and greets you warmly.

When you next see Abby, she thanks you for "not calling me out." You explain how you will behave if you see each other in public and that you will wait for her to acknowledge you. She thanks you for all your help and expresses her pride in maintaining her job and feeling better.

### Clinical Pearl: Maintaining Boundaries in a Rural Setting

In some communities, even those with larger land areas, community members may share a few public spaces in a smaller, central business district. Every situation is different, but it is entirely possible for any psychiatrist to encounter a patient (or patients) in a routine outing. Some psychiatrists prepare their patients for the moment by saying, "We need to discuss what will happen *when* we see each other in public." The reader will need to decide how to address the need for privacy—both for the reader and for the reader's patients. Some choose to live in an adjacent community, for example. Others do not have that option and must accept the fact that they may not have the luxury of refusing to see a patient because of a preexisting relationship. What happens when your child's principal has obsessive–compulsive disorder and there is no other psychiatrist for dozens of miles? Can a psychiatrist on call refuse to see a patient on consult in the community hospital because she has treated the patient's wife and the other psychiatrist in the practice is on vacation? Duty to the community may need to be weighed against duty to the individual when there is only one available psychiatrist.

## DISCUSSION

### The Art of Rural Medicine

For the purposes of this chapter, we have chosen to use the word "rural" to represent sparsely populated areas (areas with less than 2,500 residents) as well as very small and small towns (areas with between 2,500 and 49,999 residents) (US Census Bureau [USCB], n.d.). In Alabama, Arkansas, Kentucky, Montana, North Dakota, and South Dakota, between 40% and 51% of the population lives in rural areas, whereas in Maine, Mississippi, and West Virginia, greater than 51% of the population lives in rural areas (USCB, 2012). The basic techniques used in psychiatry are universally applied regardless of community size. Some special skills must be honed working in rural environments, and there are differences from working in non-rural settings. For example, systems of care models with supporting evidence in larger communities are not necessarily generalizable to rural settings: A selective serotonin reuptake inhibitor may have predictable efficacy regardless of one's residential status, but assertive community treatment is an ineffective model in underresourced areas due to the need to adapt the model to "smaller teams, less comprehensive staff, and less intensive services" (Meyer & Morrissey, 2007, p. 121). Some boundary challenges may be more easily avoided in a larger community in which it is easier to be distanced or anonymous. An outsider may be viewed as a "carpetbagger" and have trouble assimilating, whereas the same outsider in another community might be welcomed with gratitude and showers of local hospitality. Stigma is a consideration in rural settings, in part because of the "everybody-knows-my-business" phenomenon, and this may affect both patients, who can be discouraged from accessing services, and professionals, who can become discouraged about working in the setting.

### Clinical Issues

The availability of clinical services is quite variable in rural areas. In general, specialized services are more difficult to obtain, and it is reasonable to assume limited access to subspecialty psychiatrists. Child and adolescent psychiatrists, in particular, are scarce, and the rural psychiatrist may need to be comfortable treating children and adolescents. Recognizing this, some states have consultation networks in place in which a family doctor, pediatrician, or general psychiatrist can reach out to a child psychiatrist for a "curbside" or more formal consultation. Patients may need to travel great distances to access treatment. Otherwise, the services and organization of a rural community mental health center are often indistinguishable from those of urban settings. Underserved areas may have a federally qualified health center that may employ or contract with a psychiatrist to work alongside primary care and specialty providers. Nevertheless, emergency services are limited, and dedicated mental health crisis services are often unavailable.

Patients with substance use disorders living in a rural area may have an especially difficult time accessing treatment. Also, rural areas often have limited prevention resources. Geographic, political, and regional supply variables appear to drive the prevalence of one kind of substance over another, although the ubiquity of the full range of substances available in metropolitan areas should not be underestimated. Methamphetamines, illicit prescription drugs, and heroin are prevalent. Although the rates of illicit drug use are slightly less in rural areas compared to more populated areas, alcohol is a well-established problem, and underage drinking and binge drinking occur at similar rates regardless of population density. Smoking rates are higher in rural areas, and the use of smokeless tobacco is more than three times greater than in large metropolitan areas (US Department of Health and Human Services, 2014).

Suicide rates are higher in rural areas, and among youth, the suicide rate is nearly double that in urban areas and increasing (Fontanella et al., 2015). The reasons for this are speculative, but the higher rates have been attributed to access to firearms, limited service availability, and poverty. Certain groups of people who live in rural areas more than urban areas have higher rates of suicide, including Native American and Native Alaskan people, as well as military veterans (David-Ferdon, Crosby, Caine, Hindman, Reed, & Iskander, 2016).

## Culture

With every attempt to avoid overgeneralization, it is important to know that in rural communities, tradition, self-sufficiency, and hard work are values commonly expressed by the people who live there. Religion, particularly Christianity, is disproportionately practiced by residents of rural areas. Politics, of course, is complicated, but rural communities tend to be more conservative. Popular conceptions that rural areas are predominantly Caucasian are false. Some rural areas, depending on the region and local migration history, may be predominantly Hispanic, Native American, or African American, and each has its own cultural norms. Descendants of German immigrants farming the land in southern Indiana may approach situations differently than descendants of Ulster Scots working the land in Appalachia. The current representatives of the Tlingit people in Wrangell, Alaska, may view the world differently than their neighbors descended from Caucasian settlers in the 20th century, even though they share a small island with one post office and only one grocery store.

The structured culture-based interviews accompanying the DSM-5 (American Psychiatric Association, 2013) can be very helpful when entering a community with a culture unfamiliar to the practicing psychiatrist. Found on the publication's website (https://www.psychiatry.org/psychiatrists/practice/dsm), these 12 interview sets are designed to assist the clinician in cross-cultural communication (see also Chapter 4).

## Homelessness

An important factor in public psychiatry, a more detailed discussion of homelessness is provided in Chapter 19. Presenting unique challenges in the rural environment, a brief discussion of homelessness in this context is warranted.

The nature of homelessness in rural places is different than that in urban areas. Perhaps instead of sleeping in a park or on a sidewalk, one is more likely to be "couch surfing" from one living room to another. Just as rural areas cannot always afford the same health care resources found in urban areas, they often do not have resources available to combat homelessness. Frequently, individuals in rural communities do not have good access to transportation or affordable housing (National Alliance to End Homelessness [NAEH], 2015). In the United States, the larger federal housing programs target urban areas, leaving little support for less concentrated population centers (NAEH, 2015).

Despite these differences, the root cause of homelessness is likely the same in any environment: poverty and lack of access to affordable housing (NAEH, 2015). Poverty rates are higher in rural areas than in urban areas, and the median household incomes in the United States are the lowest in non-metropolitan areas (US Department of Agriculture Economic Research Service [USDA], 2012). This is due, at least in part, to lower education levels (rural areas have fewer college graduates) and fewer high-skill jobs (USDA, 2012). Prior to the Great Recession, the unemployment rate in rural areas was steadily higher than that in urban areas. This trend ceased during the recession, and as recently as 2014, the margin between metropolitan and non-metropolitan unemployment rates was much narrower. Unfortunately, this is due to a decline in the number of rural people searching for jobs, not an increase in employment (DeNavas-Walt & Proctor, 2015).

## Economics

The US Department of Agriculture (USDA, 2013) defines counties "as being persistently poor if 20% or more of their populations were living in poverty over the last 30 years." Under this definition, USCB data indicate 85% of persistently poor counties in the United States are rural (USDA, 2013). Of course, not all rural counties are persistently poor, and entire regions (e.g., New England and all of the Pacific Time Zone) have no persistently poor counties at all.

The distinct economic difference in rural places in the United States is one aspect that affects service delivery. With lower incomes and fewer jobs comes a lower tax base from which to draw upon. Distance is an additional factor, complicating the availability and expense of transportation. Although only 46.2 million US residents lived in rural counties in 2014, those residents were spread out across 72% of the country's 3.8 million square miles (USDA, 2012).

## Resources

Telemedicine has offered a recent advantage in combating the shortage of psychiatrists in rural areas. Not without limitations, including technology interfaces and reimbursement concerns, telepsychiatry is used in settings ranging from federally qualified health centers to private offices. Even the US military is using telepsychiatry to reach members and dependents attached to remote installations.

Despite the potential for rewarding work and sometimes well-compensating market opportunities, rural communities face a special challenge recruiting and maintaining a skilled workforce. Some medical schools have a rural mission and aim to train graduates with rural service in mind. Federal programs reward practice in underserved areas, and foreign medical graduates may find a warm welcome in an area that is able to sponsor special visa status.

Mid-level providers such as physician assistants and nurse practitioners have been employed successfully to supplement or extend the ability for rural patients to receive mental health care.

## REFERENCES

American Psychiatric Association. (2013). *Diagnostic and statistical manual of mental disorders* (5th ed.). Arlington, VA: American Psychiatric Publishing.

Centers for Disease Control and Prevention. (2015, April 30). *Understanding the Epidemic*. Retrieved from http://www.cdc.gov/drugoverdose/epidemic

David-Ferdon, C., Crosby, A. E., Caine, E. D., Hindman, J., Reed, J., & Iskander, J. (2016, September). CDC Grand Rounds: Preventing suicide through a comprehensive public health approach. *MMWR Morbidity and Mortality Weekly Report, 65*(34), 894–897. doi:10.15585/mmwr.mm6534a2

DeNavas-Walt, C., & Proctor, B. D. (2015, September). *Income and poverty in the United States: 2014*. Retrieved from https://www.census.gov/content/dam/Census/library/publications/2015/demo/p60-252.pdf

Fontanella, C. A., Hiance-Steelesmith, D. L., Phillips, G. S., Bridge, J. A., Lester, N., Sweeney, H. A., & Campo, J. V. (2015, May). Widening rural–urban disparities in youth suicides, United States, 1996–2010. *JAMA Pediatrics, 169*(5), 466–473. doi:10.1001/jamapediatrics.2014.3561

Fortney, J. C., Harman, J. S., Xu, S., & Dong, F. (2009, October). *Rural–urban differences in depression care*. Working paper of the Western Interstate Commission for Higher Education Mental Health Program, Boulder, CO.

Meyer, P. S., & Morrissey, J. P. (2007, January). A comparison of assertive community treatment and intensive case management for patients in rural areas. *Psychiatric Services, 58*(1), 121–127.

National Alliance to End Homelessness. (2015). *Rural homelessness*. Retrieved from http://www.endhomelessness.org/pages/rural

Syed, S. T., Gerber, B. S., & Sharp, L. K. (2013, October). Travelling towards disease: Transportation barriers to health care access. *Journal of Community Health, 38*(5), 976–993. doi:10.1007/s10900-013-9681-1

US Census Bureau. (2012, March 21). *PcturbanRural_State the spreadsheet with cited rural and urban areas (PctUrbanRural_State.xls)*. Retrieved from https://www.census.gov/geo/reference/ua/ualists_layout.html?cssp=SERP

US Census Bureau. (n.d.). *Urban and rural classification*. Retrieved from https://www.census.gov/geo/reference/urban-rural.html

US Department of Agriculture Economic Research Service. (2012, May 26). *Rural economy & population*. Retrieved from https://www.ers.usda.gov/topics/rural-economy-population.aspx

US Department of Agriculture Economic Research Service. (2013, July 19). *Persistent-poverty counties are mostly nonmetro, generally Southern.* Retrieved from https://www.ers.usda.gov/data-products/chart-gallery/gallery/chart-detail/?chartId=76826

US Department of Health and Human Services, Substance Abuse and Mental Health Services Administration, Center for Behavioral Health Statistics and Quality. (2014, September). *Results from the 2013 national survey on drug use and health: Summary of national findings.* Retrieved from https://www.samhsa.gov/data/sites/default/files/NSDUHresultsPDFWHTML2013/Web/NSDUHresults2013.pdf

Young, A. M., Havens, J. R., & Leukefeld, C. G. (2012, May). A comparison of rural and urban nonmedical prescription opioid users' lifetime and recent drug use. *American Journal of Drug and Alcohol Abuse, 38*(3), 220–227. doi:10.3109/00952990.2011.643971

# 25

# Lesbian, Gay, Bisexual, Transgender, and Queer People

## LAURA ERICKSON-SCHROTH AND ANTONIA BARBA ∎

## CASE HISTORIES

### Case 1

Josh is a 15-year-old Dominican boy who identifies as gay and lives in a residential care program for emotionally disturbed youth. Josh has limited contact with his mother, who is diagnosed with major depressive disorder and has a history of alcohol and drug abuse. Josh never lived with his father, and the last time he saw his father, Josh was 6 years old. When Josh was 10 years old, he and his sisters were removed from their mother's care due to physical abuse, and they witnessed domestic violence involving their mother and her live-in boyfriend. Her boyfriend frequently harassed Josh for his soft-spoken and shy demeanor, and he beat Josh in an effort to "toughen him up."

#### Clinical Pearl

At the age of 10 years, Josh may not yet have identified as gay or even been actively questioning his sexual orientation. Children and teens do not have to openly identify as lesbian, gay, bisexual, transgender, or queer (LGBTQ) in order to be the victims of bullying and abuse based on their gender presentation. When working with children such as Josh, it is important not to make assumptions about sexual orientation based solely on external presentation.

The children lived in a series of foster homes before being placed in the guardianship of their maternal grandmother. While in foster care, Josh was sexually abused by another child in the home and also experienced ongoing bullying and social isolation at school. He began receiving supportive counseling, and it was recommended that he start trauma-focused therapy to help him with his emerging symptoms of anxiety and depression. Eligibility and access to treatment changed after his grandmother's guardianship was formalized, and he discontinued treatment.

Josh struggled to adjust to life in his new home. His grandmother found him very changed from the sweet young boy he had been and began to focus her attention on Josh's sisters, for whom she felt better able to care. Josh became more withdrawn and increasingly irritable, with incidents of volatile and destructive behavior, often yelling, slamming doors, and throwing objects. By the age of 13 years, these behaviors had escalated to the point that he required hospitalization, followed by an 8-month stay in a residential treatment facility. While there, he was frequently teased and bullied by his peers because he was perceived as gay. Program staff witnessed this verbal and occasionally physical abuse but rarely intervened. His depression and aggression intensified, and he was hospitalized after experiencing active suicidal ideation.

**Clinical Pearl**

When working with LGBTQ youth who have experienced abuse and disrupted attachments, it is critical to recognize the resulting behavioral health problems as sequelae of trauma and not a consequence of being LGBTQ. LGBTQ youth may be more vulnerable to experiencing trauma and abuse, but this is largely due to external factors and not inherent pathology. However, LGBTQ identity and trauma may be connected in the mind of the client, particularly in the case of sexual abuse. Children can have a number of troubling reactions, including fear that their sexual orientation somehow caused them to be abused or confusion about whether the abuse was really abuse. LGBTQ youth may be hesitant to report abuse due to fear that they will be outed or labeled as sexual predators. In this case, Josh's symptoms can be considered a normative response to the chronic abuse he has experienced.

Josh arrives at your program with a diagnosis of major depressive disorder and intermittent explosive disorder (IED) and is taking sertraline and risperidone to address his depressive symptoms and aggressive behaviors. He forms a positive relationship with his therapist and is generally well regarded by his residential counselors, but he struggles to engage socially with his peers. His counselors state that he is often moody and argumentative, and they think he is hypersensitive and too easily takes offense. After evaluating him and learning about the extent of his abuse history, you change his diagnosis to remove IED and include post-traumatic stress disorder (PTSD), and you speak to Josh about beginning a course of trauma treatment with his therapist. Josh is reluctant to talk about the abuse and blames himself for it. He is mistrustful of the program and his fellow residents, and he tells you that he feels unsafe. He does agree to attend weekly therapy sessions and to learn more about trauma-focused therapy.

## Case 2

Ms. Johnson is a 28-year-old African American transgender woman (MTF) living by herself in Section 8 housing, supporting herself on public assistance and food stamps, with an application submitted for Supplemental Security Income. She grew up in North Carolina and moved to Washington, DC, at age 17 years when she was kicked out of her grandmother's house for dressing in female clothing.

### Clinical Pearl

Transgender women are those who are assigned male at birth and identify as female, also known as the more medicalized term male-to-female (MTF), whereas transgender men are those who are assigned female at birth and identify as male, also known as female-to-male (FTM). Although few people self-identify using the abbreviations MTF or FTM, these can be useful when communicating with colleagues who are less familiar with transgender identities.

Questions regarding hormonal or surgical history may be asked at the appropriate times during the initial interview (i.e., when discussing current medications or during the medical/surgical history). If you are talking to another provider about a transgender client, the client's history of hormone use or surgeries is often irrelevant to the issue being discussed, in which case there is no need to bring it up.

Because she never finished high school, it has been difficult for Ms. Johnson to find a job, and she has been in and out of jail and prison for nonviolent charges, including solicitation and drug sales. She has a history of heavy alcohol and marijuana use in her early 20s, but she has been sober since going to prison for 2 years from ages 23 to 25 years. Although her substance abuse is in remission, since being in prison, she developed other psychiatric issues.

Prior to going to prison, Ms. Johnson had never sought professional help, and she remembers having some short periods of depression, with intermittent thoughts of suicide but never any attempts. She was sent to a men's prison upstate, where she suffered innumerable abuses from both other inmates and guards, and she spent an entire year in solitary confinement, ostensibly for her own safety. In solitary, she began to hear voices, which transformed into command auditory hallucinations to kill herself. She tried to commit suicide twice—once by hanging herself with her bed sheets and the other time by cutting her wrist with a plastic fork.

Ms. Johnson received mental health services in prison, but not until the last few months she was there, after she made a suicide attempt. After she was released, she began to see a community psychiatrist and started quetiapine and weekly supportive therapy. She decided to seek legal help to sue the state for the abuses she had suffered in prison. She eventually completed treatment and was doing very well until she began to work on her deposition with her lawyer and had to spend time recalling the events that had happened to her. This process led to a return of nightmares, increased startle response, and auditory hallucinations. At this point, she presented to the clinic where you work, asking for quetiapine and for a letter to give the judge in her case, requesting accommodations for her mental illness.

### Clinical Pearl

Hormonal regimens for transgender individuals—which usually include testosterone for transgender men and estrogen plus an androgen blocker such as spironolactone for transgender women—generally do not induce psychiatric issues such as anxiety or depression. Many transgender people report improvement in depression and anxiety symptoms after beginning hormones. Be aware of any drug–drug interactions between the client's hormone treatments and any other medications. For example, lithium should be used very cautiously in a client on spironolactone because the combination can increase lithium to dangerous levels. As in pregnancy, lamotrigine doses may need to be increased significantly to reach the same blood levels if a client is on estrogen.

After evaluating her, you tell Ms. Johnson that you can write a letter for her explaining to the judge that you believe she meets criteria for PTSD and asking that she have access to available services. You then discuss treatment for PTSD, explaining that psychotherapy and selective serotonin reuptake inhibitors are first line. She voices an understanding but says that quetiapine has been helpful for her in the past, and she feels very vulnerable right now. You check with her about other medications she is on (only estrogen and spironolactone) and agree to restart quetiapine and supportive therapy and revisit medication options later.

## DISCUSSION

### LGBTQ Terminology

*Gender identity* refers to one's inner sense of self as male, female, both, or neither. The terms *cisgender* and *transgender* describe individuals whose gender identity and sex assigned at birth are congruent or not congruent, respectively. Transgender is an umbrella term that can cover a broad range of identities, including those who identify as genderqueer or androgynous. There are many people who believe the gender binary is restrictive and view themselves as living in between genders or possessing traits consistent with both genders. Gender expression refers to the outward expression or presentation of one's gender and can include attire and demeanor. An individual's gender expression may or may not be congruent with the individual's gender identity. Environment, safety considerations, and pressures to adapt or conform are among factors determining gender expression choices. Some transgender people are interested in taking hormones or having surgeries, whereas others are not. There are various reasons why some people choose to take certain steps to socially and/or medically transition. Finances can play a major role; most health care plans do not currently cover transition-related care. Decisions can also be influenced by social and relationship situations, sexual functioning, and attainable aesthetic.

*Sexual orientation* describes a person's pattern of attraction. Because the terms straight, gay, or bisexual assume that gender is binary, many people identify as pansexual if they have the potential to be attracted to people of all genders, including transgender and genderqueer people. An individual's sexual self-identification is not necessarily indicative of the individual's behavior.

LGBTQ terminology can depend on culture, race, and ethnicity. Native American cultures may refer to transgender people as Two-Spirit. Transgender Latina women may call themselves translatinas. It is common in some African

American communities for people to refer to themselves as men or women "of transgender experience" rather than as transgender people.

## Trauma, Violence, and Minority Stress Theory

LGBTQ populations have a high burden of trauma. A history of harassment, discrimination, victimization, violence, or forced sex is reported by 50–80% of transgender people studied (Carmel, Hopwood, & Dickey, 2014). The unemployment rate of transgender people is twice as high as that of the general public (Grant et al., 2011). Race and ethnicity may affect risk for trauma: 67% of LGBTQ homicide victims are transgender women of color (Ahmed & Jindasurat, 2014).

LGBTQ youth experience higher rates of emotional and physical abuse, bullying, and dating violence compared to their peers (Centers for Disease Control and Prevention, 2011). These factors place them at risk for developing depression, suicidal ideation and attempts, illegal drug use, and high-risk sexual behaviors (Ryan, Huebner, Diaz, & Sanchez, 2009). Members of other marginalized groups are often able to draw strength from within their families based on shared experiences of stigma and discrimination. Because sexual orientation and gender identity are not shared family traits, LGBTQ youth often do not receive this same type of support, which further increases their isolation.

The minority stress model predicts that minority groups experience stress related to identity-based stigmatization and discrimination, resulting in negative mental health outcomes (Meyer, 1995). There is evidence that due to minority stress, LGBTQ people have increased rates of depression, substance abuse, self-harm, and suicidality (Carmel et al., 2014).

A small but burgeoning field in LGBTQ studies revolves around resilience-building. Social and family support appear to be two very important factors in promoting resilience under difficult circumstances (Ryan, Russell, Huebner, Diaz, & Sanchez, 2010). Navigating trauma may arm some individuals with effective coping skills and nontraditional sources of support.

## LGBTQ People and Psychiatry

LGBTQ people have a long and complicated history with the field of psychiatry, affecting how they approach mental health care. Due to a legacy of pathologization, as well as attempts at reparative or conversion therapy, many LGBTQ people avoid mental health providers entirely. When forced to interact with psychiatrists to gain clearance for medical or surgical interventions, many transgender people view psychiatrists as gatekeepers and often believe they have to present a specific narrative in order to be given access to these interventions.

Psychiatry pathologized homosexuality long before the publication of DSM-I in 1952. Eventually, activists were able to push for debates within the American Psychiatric Association, which led to the removal of homosexuality as a diagnosis in 1973. A diagnosis of "ego-dystonic homosexuality" remained until 1987.

DSM-III, in 1980, included gender identity disorder, which survives as gender dysphoria in DSM-5 today (Drescher, 2010).

## LGBTQ-Affirmative Care

Psychiatrists and mental health programs can provide welcoming environments by decorating with LGBTQ-affirming posters, hiring sensitive front desk staff, providing staff and community education, utilizing LGBTQ-inclusive intake forms, and making gender-neutral restrooms easily accessible.

Respectful history-taking includes open-ended questions about gender identity and sexual orientation. This may include using the term "partner(s)" in place of gendered terms when inquiring about a client's relationships and also asking clients to describe their gender or sexual orientation rather than making assumptions. If clients do not volunteer information about the pronouns (i.e., he, she, they, etc.) or name they use, it is important to ask and then to use these when speaking with or about the client.

## LGBTQ People with Serious and Persistent Mental Illness

Bipolar disorder and schizophrenia prevalence is not increased among LGBTQ people. However, LGBTQ people with these serious mental illnesses (SMI) often have difficulty finding affirmative care, and they may be ostracized from LGBTQ communities at the same time. Historically, sexual and gender minorities have been labeled psychotic for their beliefs about their identities. People with SMI may present with gender- or sexuality-related themes in the context of psychosis or mania that make it difficult for clinicians to distinguish between identity and illness. This can complicate assessment of the appropriateness of hormonal or surgical interventions. Clinicians should support clients in establishing a sense of who they are when they are well. In addition, many clinicians view people with SMI as too sick to have sexual lives. Like most other people, people with SMI benefit from close connections, and they should be encouraged to develop safe and respectful romantic relationships.

Inpatient and residential programs may have regulatory requirements to provide safe spaces for LGBTQ individuals, but they often lack the knowledge and resources to provide much beyond superficial accommodations. These programs are generally arranged on a gender binary system with men's and women's dorms and bathrooms. Transgender and gender nonconforming people who do not easily fit into this system pose challenges for, and may even experience hostility from, program staff and peers, causing them to feel unwelcome and unsafe (Lucksted, 2004).

LGBTQ individuals who have experienced subtle or overt stigma may benefit from programs specifically designed to meet their needs. Many specialized organizations began as grassroots and volunteer-staffed initiatives. For example, Boston's Fenway Community Health, one of 14 LGBTQ health centers in the United States, began as a neighborhood clinic and has matured into a model of care that includes primary, specialty, and integrated behavioral health services and a range of wellness programs. This organization has established standards for LGBTQ cultural responsiveness and promotes community-based research and a robust professional educational program. Research on the effectiveness of LGBTQ-specialized programs is limited, but, as is discussed elsewhere in this volume, culturally responsive services support engagement and treatment adherence.

Psychiatrists who are open to learning about LGBTQ individuals and communities can help address some of the mental health disparities that result from discrimination. They can assist LGBTQ people in building resilience, and be part of the development of an equitable and just society.

## REFERENCES

Ahmed, O., & Jindasurat, C. (2014). *Lesbian, gay, bisexual, transgender, queer and HIV-affected hate violence in 2013*. New York, NY: National Coalition of Anti-Violence Programs.

Carmel, T., Hopwood, R., & Dickey, L. (2014). Mental health concerns. In L. Erickson-Schroth (Ed.), *Trans bodies, trans selves: A resource guide for the transgender community* (pp. 305–332). New York, NY: Oxford University Press.

Centers for Disease Control and Prevention. (2011). Sexual identity, sex of sexual contacts, and health-risk behaviors among students in grades 9–12: Youth Risk Behavior Surveillance, selected sites, United States, 2001–2009. *MMMR Morbidity and Mortality Weekly Report: Surveillance Summaries, 60*(7), 1–133.

Drescher, J. (2010). Queer diagnoses: Parallels and contrasts in the history of homosexuality, gender variance, and the *Diagnostic and Statistical Manual. Archives of Sexual Behavior, 39*(2), 427–460.

Grant, J. M., Mottet, L., Tanis, J. E., Harrison, J., Herman, J., & Keisling, M. (2011). *Injustice at every turn: A report of the National Transgender Discrimination Survey.* Washington, DC: National Center for Transgender Equality.

Lucksted, A. (2004). Raising issues: Lesbian, gay, bisexual & transgender people receiving services in the public mental health system. *Journal of Gay & Lesbian Mental Health, 8*(3–4), 25–42.

Meyer, I. H. (1995). Minority stress and mental health in gay men. *Journal of Health and Social Behavior, 36*, 38–56.

Ryan, C., Huebner, D., Diaz, R. M., & Sanchez, J. (2009). Family rejection as a predictor of negative health outcomes in White and Latino lesbian, gay, and bisexual young adults. *Pediatrics, 123*, 346–352.

Ryan, C., Russell, S. T., Huebner, D., Diaz, R., & Sanchez, J. (2010). Family acceptance in adolescence and the health of LGBT young adults. *Journal of Child and Adolescent Psychiatric Nursing, 23*(4), 205–213.

# 26

# Veterans

GERTIE QUITANGON ■

To care for he who shall have borne the battle.

*—Abraham Lincoln*

## CASE HISTORY

Trevor is a 25-year-old married man from the South who is looking for work in New York City a year after the end of his tour of duty in Afghanistan. He held off plans to pursue a degree in social work until after his wife completes Teachers College. Then he heard about the Veterans Integration to Academic Leadership (VITAL) initiative from a fellow veteran, and he met a VITAL coordinator who signed him up for a work-study program through the Post-9/11 GI Bill. She also connected him to an Operation Iraqi Freedom/Operation Enduring Freedom/Operation New Dawn (OEF/OIF/OND) case manager and set up a primary care appointment at the US Department of Veterans Affairs (VA) medical center. He is subsequently referred by his case manager to your community-based outpatient clinic (CBOC) in Brooklyn for further assessment of sleep difficulties.

### Clinical Pearl

The VA system is vast and complex and can be daunting for veterans and providers alike. Veterans of the recent wars are typically assigned to an OIF/OEF/OND readjustment services case manager to assist them in navigating the VA system. Having a point person who can direct the veteran to appropriate resources—from VA benefits counseling to referral for employment and linkages to health care services in a VA facility or programs in the community—helps diminish barriers and enhance service delivery to these veterans.

The Servicemen's Readjustment Act of 1944, more popularly known as the GI bill, expanded veterans' benefits to include financial assistance for education and a monthly housing allowance. After World War II, approximately 8 million veterans participated in an education or training program through the GI Bill (US Department of Veterans Affairs, 2015b). The bill was updated in August 2009 after the September 11 terrorist attacks and is now called the Post-9/11 GI bill.

The VITAL initiative is a partnership between the VA health care system and local colleges and universities. Their goal is to reach out to veterans in school settings and assist them in their transition from soldier to student. VITAL offers work-study opportunities, free tutoring, advocacy, and counseling for issues unique to veterans that could impact their performance and academic success.

Trevor requested referral to a CBOC because of its proximity to his residence. Geographic distance is a significant barrier to health care in states in which some veterans live hours away from a VA medical center, and sometimes a CBOC is their only option for access to health care. In places where veterans live more than 40 miles from the closest VA facility, the Veterans Access, Choice, and Accountability Act of 2014 ("the Choice Act") gives veterans the option to receive health care services from a non-VA provider.

Your primary care colleague performed a physical exam including a traumatic brain injury (TBI) screen, on which Trevor screened positive. A consult was then sent to the TBI clinic for further evaluation. His post-traumatic stress disorder (PTSD) screen was negative.

### Clinical Pearl

Veterans seen at the VA are followed by a primary care provider (PCP) and a patient aligned care team (PACT), the VA's team-based model of primary care. In order to best determine who is in need of further evaluation, the use of screening tools known as *clinical reminders*, such as the TBI and PTSD screens, has been a standard of practice in the VA health care system (Rathmell et al., 2012). All VA service providers are prompted to complete periodic clinical reminders during each visit, and veterans are referred for appropriate interventions when necessary. Some screening tools specific to mental health include the suicide screen, PTSD screen (Primary Care PTSD screen [PC-PTSD]), evaluation for abnormal involuntary movements scale (Abnormal Involuntary Movements Scale [AIMS]), depression screen (Patient Health Questionnaire-2 [PHQ-2]), and alcohol screen (Alcohol Use Disorders Identification Test [AUDIT-C]).

Trevor tells you that insomnia is the most distressing symptom for him. His PCP had prescribed trazodone, which helped. You assess his sleep hygiene, and he describes a significant history of alcohol use, which escalated after deployment, but he denies drinking alcohol since he moved to New York because he cannot afford it. He denies illicit drug use. His father was a heavy drinker who died of complications of liver cirrhosis. There is no other history of mental illness in his family.

Although the PTSD screen completed by his PCP was negative, you review the symptoms with him and learn that he is irritable and has difficulty concentrating, always feeling on edge and unable to relax at home. He describes how challenging the move to Brooklyn has been. "We have no space . . . the apartment is so small . . . it's so expensive . . . and my wife and I are fighting about everything," he laments. You explore his social supports. He discloses the death of two good friends by suicide this past year. You spend some time processing his thoughts and feelings about the death of his friends and assess safety issues. He adamantly denies suicidal or homicidal thoughts, then pauses and reflects, "I think about my funeral. . . . I don't think of killing myself or anything like that but I find myself visualizing the details . . . what I wear . . . the flowers . . . the music playing . . . who's going to be there . . ." as his eyes well up.

You validate his feelings and explore his service history and military trauma exposure. Trevor served in the United States Marine Corps, H&S Battalion, Provisional Rifle Company. As a gunner in a Humvee, Trevor was deployed in Afghanistan 8 months and recounts several experiences in which he believed his life was in danger. Once, he hit his head on the gun handles when his vehicle was ambushed and the driver hit the brakes abruptly. He denies loss of consciousness or any significant post-concussive symptoms, but he had transient disorientation, confusion, and blurry vision. He did not seek medical attention at that time. He also reports exposure to multiple improvised explosive devices (IEDs) and mortar blasts, but he denies any associated head trauma. He endorses witnessing and learning of several deaths during deployment that remain on his mind.

### Clinical Pearl

Not all combat trauma patients present with classic symptoms of PTSD or screen positive. It was the OIF/OEF/OND case manager who referred him for further mental health evaluation, illustrating the benefit of having a case manager who can engage veterans who otherwise may not seek appropriate interventions.

Traumatic brain injury has been considered the signature injury of the modern wars, typically caused by blast waves from IEDs or rocket-propelled grenades (Martin et al., 2009). The majority of TBI cases are mild, commonly known as concussions, usually characterized by a limited duration of loss of consciousness and post-traumatic amnesia. Treatment is supportive, and the expected recovery to premorbid functioning is variable, between 1 month to 1 year from the time of injury. Those with more severe TBI are referred for formal neuropsychiatric testing, functional evaluation, or cognitive remediation (Spelman, Hunt, Seal, & Burgo-Black, 2012).

Trevor presents as a personable young man, initially apprehensive but later fully engaged in the interview. There is no evidence of psychosis, mania, or gross cognitive deficits.

You provide feedback on insomnia, alcohol use, and PTSD symptoms and recommend individual and group treatment options. Trevor expresses interest in attending a weekly OIF/OEF/OND support group, but at this time he only wishes to continue trazodone for insomnia. You discuss potential side effects and ask him to return to the clinic in 1 month.

You process his thoughts about death and a sense of foreshortened future. You also discuss the increased risk of suicide among veterans and offer support should he have suicidal thoughts in the future. You provide your contact information and also information about the Veterans Crisis Line (phone: 1-800-273-8255; website: https://www.veteranscrisisline.net; or text: 838255).

**Clinical Pearl**

The risk for suicide for veterans is 21% higher than that for non-veterans (US Department of Veterans Affairs, 2016). It is important to note that not all military veterans served in combat, so factors affecting the increasing suicide rate in the general population may be reflected among veterans as well. According to the Centers for Disease Control and Prevention (CDC), the suicide rate in the general population has been steadily increasing since 1999, and it was the 10th leading cause of death in the United States in 2014 (Curtin, Warner, & Hedegaard, 2016).

VA efforts to address veteran suicide include the creation of the National Veterans Suicide Prevention Hotline in 2007 (renamed the Veterans Crisis Line in 2011), designation of centers focused on suicide research (i.e., the Mental Illness Research Education and Clinical Center [MIRECC] and the Center of Excellence), and establishment of the VA Suicide Prevention Program and suicide prevention coordinators (SPCs). Each VA facility has SPCs who provide an added layer of support for both veterans and mental health clinicians, and together they develop a safety plan for veterans identified as being at high risk for suicide. SPCs also raise awareness about the program and other behavioral health resources in the community.

Trevor returns for follow-up 1 month later. During the 4th of July, he reports drinking heavily with a buddy who was in town. He was distressed to learn that a third friend had committed suicide. "He shot himself . . . he was never deployed . . . had a rocky relationship and broke up with this girl not long ago," he rambles. Trevor reports that the July 4th fireworks made him feel jumpy and triggered unwanted memories of his service. He has not slept well, taking only half the dose of trazodone because he was worried about priapism. He finds himself isolating and feels emotionally detached from his wife. Their arguments have escalated. He denies being physically aggressive, but he worries about losing control at times. He continues to have detailed thoughts of his funeral, and feels like he does not have a future. He denies nightmares or flashbacks of military experiences.

You and Trevor discuss the factors contributing to his alcohol use and the risks associated with it. You discuss medication options, including antidepressants to help with PTSD symptoms. You recommend psychotherapy and discuss VA resources. You suggest meeting with him and his wife during the next visit to obtain collateral information and explore referrals for couples counseling. Trevor is ambivalent about taking medications but agrees to take the full dose of trazodone and try individual psychotherapy and the weekly OIF/OEF/OND support group.

## DISCUSSION

The VA is the second largest federal department in the United States and is responsible for providing services and benefits to America's military veterans. It is composed of a VA Central Office in Washington, DC, and three organizations: the

Veterans Health Administration(VHA), the Veterans Benefits Administration, and the National Cemetery Administration. The VHA is the largest of the three VA administrations and is also the largest, nationally integrated, publicly funded health care system in the country. Its 150 medical centers and 819 CBOCs provide medical, surgical, rehabilitative, and mental health care to approximately 8 million veterans, and it is a major training ground for medical, nursing, and allied health professionals in the United States (Gordon, 2015).

Dating as far back as the return of the Vietnam War veterans, the VA has struggled to overcome organizational challenges and controversies. The media's tendency to highlight long wait lists and other systemic issues has overshadowed the VA's contribution to education, research, and innovation. In the field of mental health, the VA has been pioneering advances in the evaluation and treatment of PTSD and TBI.

The VA delivers comprehensive services to a vulnerable population—older, indigent, and many with combat-related injuries—yet a study showed that the VA is more cost-effective than the private sector across the range of inpatient, outpatient, and prescription drug services (Busch, Leslie, & Rosenheck, 2004). Another study comparing process-based quality outcomes in the evaluation and management of mental health and substance use disorders revealed that the quality of care provided at the VA far exceeded that of the private sector (Watkins et al., 2016). Based on findings of cost-effectiveness and high-quality care, the current health care system for veterans can be considered a model for universal health care for all Americans.

Mental health care for veterans has evolved considerably from World War I to the post-9/11 era. The experience of the Vietnam War veterans first brought attention to the phenomenology of PTSD, and now there are multiple PTSD treatment modalities supported by research evidence. Approximately 500,000 veterans of the Iraq and Afghanistan conflicts who receive care through the VA have been diagnosed with potential or provisional PTSD (US Department of Veterans Affairs, 2015c). The three most common diagnoses of veterans from these conflicts were musculoskeletal diseases, mental disorders, and "symptoms, signs and ill-defined condition," suggesting that many more veterans may present a broader post-traumatic syndrome. (US Department of Veterans Affairs, 2015a).

Among veterans who seek care at the VA, 1 in 4 women and 1 in 100 men reported that they experienced military sexual trauma (MST) (US Department of Veterans Affairs, 2017a). MST is defined as psychological trauma from sexual assault or sexual harassment that occurred during service (Federal Law Title 38 US Code 1720D), and it has been associated with an increased risk of PTSD, mood and anxiety disorders, as well as substance abuse (Kimerling et al., 2007). The MST program at the VA includes having an MST coordinator at each facility and mandatory training for mental health and primary care providers on MST screening and other MST-related issues. Residential and inpatient treatment specializing in sexual trauma is available for those who need a higher level of care.

1 in 10 Iraq and Afghanistan veterans seen at the VA report alcohol or drug misuse (US Department of Veterans Affairs, 2017b). The co-occurrence of PTSD and substance use disorder (SUD) both in civilian and in military populations is well known, and among veterans, 2 out of 10 diagnosed with PTSD also have SUD (US Department of Veterans Affairs, 2017b). The VA offers short- and long-term inpatient and outpatient treatment programming for both PTSD and SUD. It also has an employment program called Compensated Work Therapy–Transitional Work

Experience (CWT-TWE), which is designed for veterans recovering from chemical dependency, many of whom have a history of PTSD and homelessness.

The VA has had remarkable success in providing housing and comprehensive medical, psychiatric, and case management services for homeless veterans delivered by specialized programs such as Housing and Urban Development VA Supportive Housing (HUD-VASH), Homeless-Patient Aligned Care Team (H-PACT), and Housing First ACT (assertive community treatment) team. In 2014, the VA launched trauma-informed care (TIC) for homeless veterans to address the connection between homelessness and trauma exposure and PTSD (US Department of Veterans Affairs, 2017c). Health care providers are trained to screen for PTSD in homeless veterans in order to reduce barriers to care and create a trauma-informed environment conducive to their recovery.

The Veterans Affairs/Department of Defense's (VA/DOD) *Clinical Practice Guidelines for the Management of Post-Traumatic Stress* (2010) recommended either medication or psychotherapy as first-line treatment for those who meet criteria for PTSD, those who have significant symptoms suggestive of PTSD, or those with functional impairment. The guidelines recommend selective serotonin and noradrenaline reuptake inhibitors as first-line medications, whereas mirtazapine, prazosin, tricyclic antidepressants, and monoamine oxidase inhibitors are second line. Of note, benzodiazepines have not been found to be effective in clinical trials and are not recommended.

Major PTSD treatment guidelines recommend exposure-based psychotherapy and cognitive–behavioral approaches (Wolfe, 2015). The VA has implemented a large-scale initiative to disseminate the use of individual and group prolonged exposure therapy and cognitive processing therapy, as well as other evidence-based psychotherapeutic interventions including acceptance and commitment therapy and Skills Training and Affect Regulation (Rathmell et al., 2012). Adjunctive services and alternative treatment approaches recommended by the VA/DOD guidelines, including spiritual support and acupuncture, are also widely available at VA facilities.

Because of the high rates of mental illness and disability in the veteran population, improvement of mental health care has been a VA institutional priority. This chapter illustrates some of the structures and programs designed to overcome barriers and enhance access to the delivery of evidence-informed mental health practices at the VA.


## ACKNOWLEDGEMENT

Special thanks to Richard J. Pinard, LCSW-R, Transition Care (OEF/OIF/OND) Program Manager at the VA NY Harbor Healthcare System for his invaluable contribution to this chapter.


## REFERENCES

Busch, S. H., Leslie, D. L., & Rosenheck, R. A. (2004). Comparing the quality of antidepressant pharmacotherapy in the Department of Veterans Affairs and the private sector. *Psychiatric Services, 55,* 1386–1391.

Curtin, S. C., Warner, M., & Hedegaard, H. (2016). *Increase in suicide in the United States, 1999–2014* (NCHS data brief No. 241). Hyattsville, MD: National Center for Health Statistics.

Gordon, S. (2015, Fall). Unfriendly fire: Despite ideological attacks and under-funding, the Veterans Health Administration is a model public system. *The American Prospect*. Retrieved from http://prospect.org/article/why-veterans-health-system-better-you-think

Kimerling, R., Gima, K., Smith, M. W., Street, A., & Frayne, S. (2007). The Veterans Health Administration and military sexual trauma. *American Journal of Public Health, 97*, 2160–2166.

Martin, M., Oh, J., Currier, H., Beekley, A., Eckert, M., & Holcomb, J. (2009). An analysis of in-hospital deaths at a modern combat support hospital. *Journal of Trauma, 66*(4 Suppl.), S51–S61.

Rathmell, S. R., Ryan, W. G., Isbill, S. D., Norton, M. J., Foster, K. R., Metz, G., & Kennemer, D. L. (2012). Veterans and war. In H. L. McQuistion, W. E. Sowers, J. M. Ranz, & J. M. Feldman (Eds.), *Handbook of community psychiatry* (pp. 447–457). New York, NY: Springer.

Spelman, J. F., Hunt, S. C., Seal, K. H., & Burgo-Black, A. L. (2012). Post deployment care for returning combat veterans. *Journal of General Internal Medicine, 27*(9), 1200-1209.

US Department of Veterans Affairs & US Department of Defense. (2010). Management of post-traumatic stress disorder and acute stress reaction. In *VA/DoD clinical practice guideline for the management of post-traumatic stress* (pp. 58–95). Washington, DC. US Department of Veterans Affairs.

US Department of Veterans Affairs. (2015a). *Analysis of VA health care utilization among Operation Enduring Freedom (OEF), Operation Iraqi Freedom (OIF), and Operation New Dawn (OND) Veterans: From 1st Qtr FY 2002 through 2nd Qtr FY 2015*. Retrieved from https://www.publichealth.va.gov/docs/epidemiology/healthcare-utilization-report-fy2014-qtr1.pdf

US Department of Veterans Affairs. (2015b). *Benefits and eligibility*. Retrieved from https://www.benefits.va.gov/gibill

US Department of Veterans Affairs. (2015c). *Report on VA facility specific Operation Enduring Freedom (OEF), Operation Iraqi Freedom (OIF), and Operation New Dawn (OND) veterans diagnosed with potential or provisional PTSD: From 1st Qtr FY 2002 through 2nd Qtr FY 2015*. Retrieved from https://www.publichealth.va.gov/docs/epidemiology/ptsd-report-fy2015-qtr1.pdf

US Department of Veterans Affairs, Office of Suicide Prevention. (2016). *Suicide among veterans and other Americans: 2001–2014*. Retrieved from https://www.mental-health.va.gov/docs/2016suicidedatareport.pdf 10/7/2016

US Department of Veterans Affairs. (2017a). *Military sexual trauma*. Retrieved from https://www.ptsd.va.gov/public/types/violence/military-sexual-trauma-general.asp

US Department of Veterans Affairs. (2017b). *PTSD and substance abuse in veterans*. Retrieved from https://www.ptsd.va.gov/public/problems/ptsd_substance_abuse_veterans.asp

US Department of Veterans Affairs. (2017c). *Trauma-informed care: Awareness and education in homeless programs*. Retrieved from https://www.va.gov/homeless/nchav/education/trauma-informed-care.asp

Watkins, K. E., Smith, B., Akincigil, A., Sorbero, M. E., Paddock, S., Woodroffe, A., . . . Pincus, H. A. (2016). The quality of medication treatment for mental disorders in the Department of Veterans Affairs and in private-sector plans. *Psychiatric Services, 67*(4), 391–396.

Wolfe, J. P. (2015). *Using meta-analysis to determine the most effective treatments for post-traumatic stress disorder.* Retrieved from http://www.dcoe.mil/training/webinars/2015/using-meta-analysis-determine-most-effective-treatments-posttraumatic-stress-disorder

Tables, figures, and boxes are indicated by an italic *t*, *f*, or *b* following the page number.